Keto Chaffle and Intermittent Fasting

2 Books in 1

Start Your day With Delicious Keto Chaffle Recipes and Through Intermittent Fasting Lose Weight, Heal Your Body and Supercharge Your Health

By

Zoe Nelson

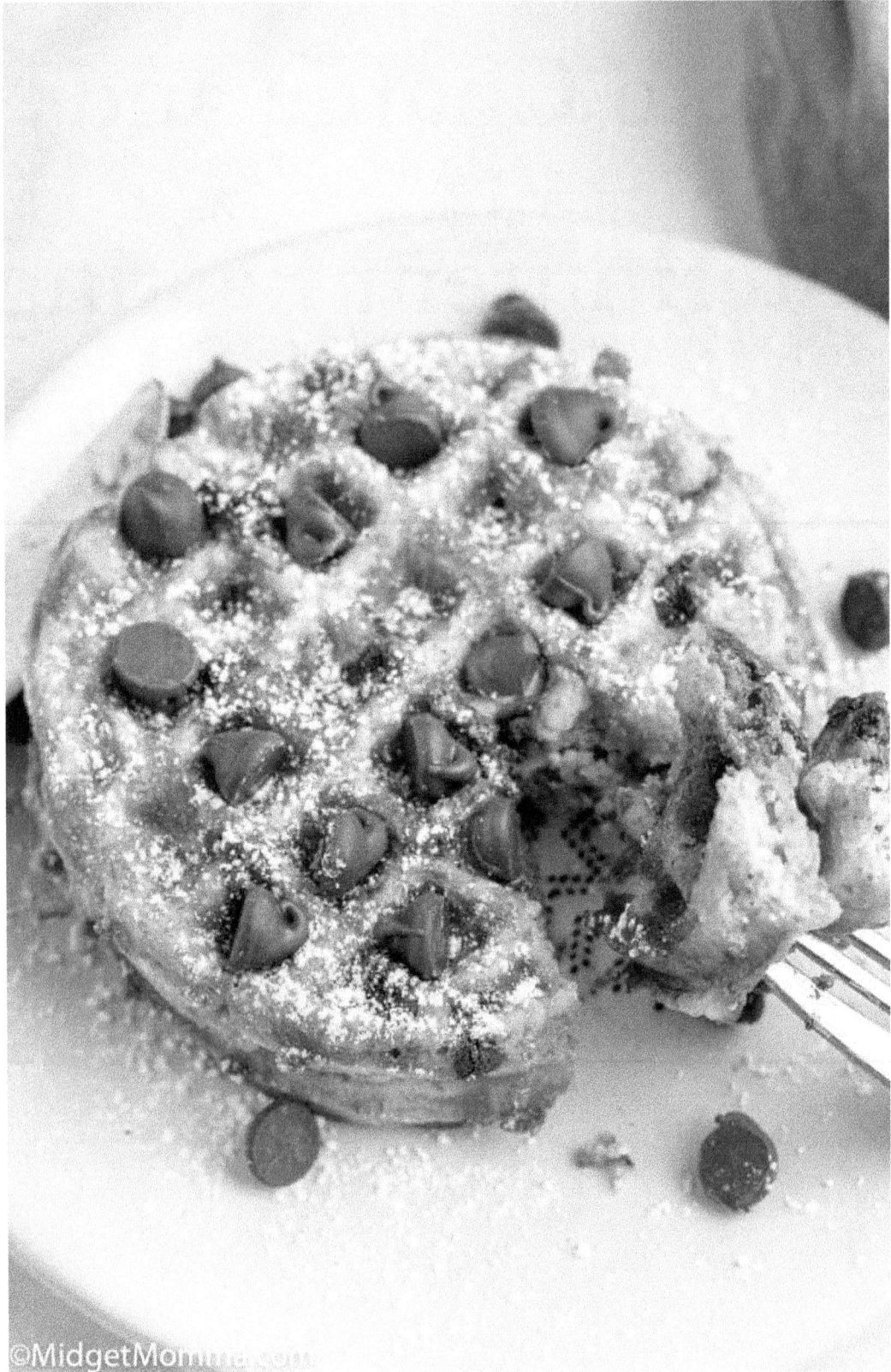

TABLE OF CONTENTS

INTERMITTENT FASTING AND KETO DIET

KETO CHAFFLE COOKBOOK

Intermittent Fasting and Keto diet

A Complete Plan Diet To Recharge Your Metabolism and Heal Your Body With Delicious Recipes To make At Home.

By

Zoe Nelson

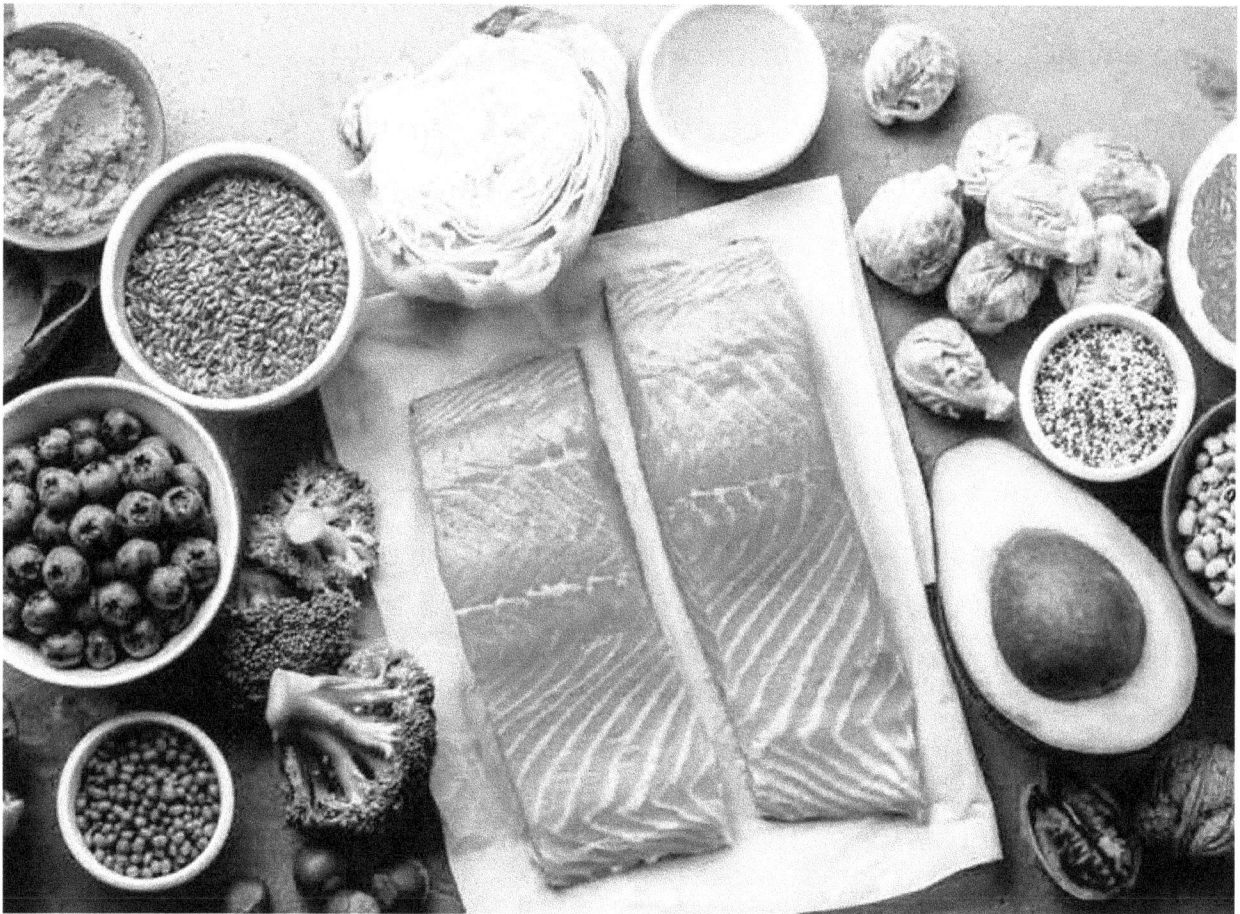

INTRODUCTION

Congratulations on purchasing Keto and intermittent fasting: Your Essential Guide for a Low-Carb Diet for Perfect Mind-Body Balance, Weight Loss, With Ketogenic Recipes to Maximize Your Health and thank you for doing so.

We really hope that you are able to get the most benefit of this book since it was made with a lot of effort and willingness to help people to improve their health, lose weight or overcome any of the problems that the keto diet can help with.

In the following chapters, you will be able to find tons of really interesting information, starting from scratch, about the keto diet, how it works, benefits, risks, fasting, autophagy, how to relate both keto and intermittent fasting and many other awesome facts that will help you to change your lifestyle, starting from your feeding habits.

The chapters here written will teach you everything you need to know about the Ketogenic diet, the state of ketosis, which foods are allowed when following keto diet, fasting and different types of fasting, how to know if I am able to stick to this diet, why does people stress and how will this diet help about it, mental improvements, and many many other extraordinary information.

There are plenty of books on this subject on the market, thanks again for choosing this one! Every effort was made to ensure it is full of as much useful information as possible; please enjoy!

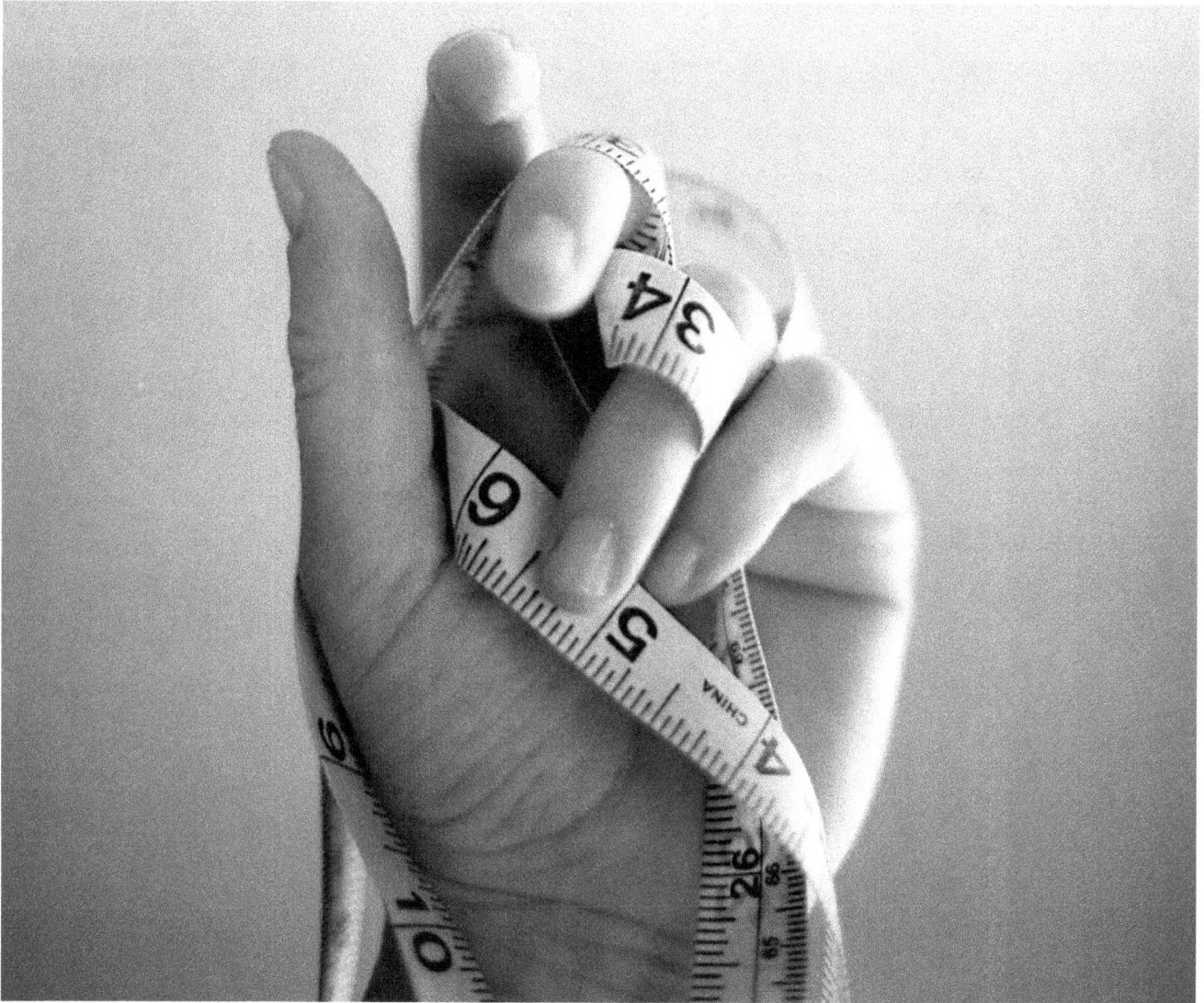

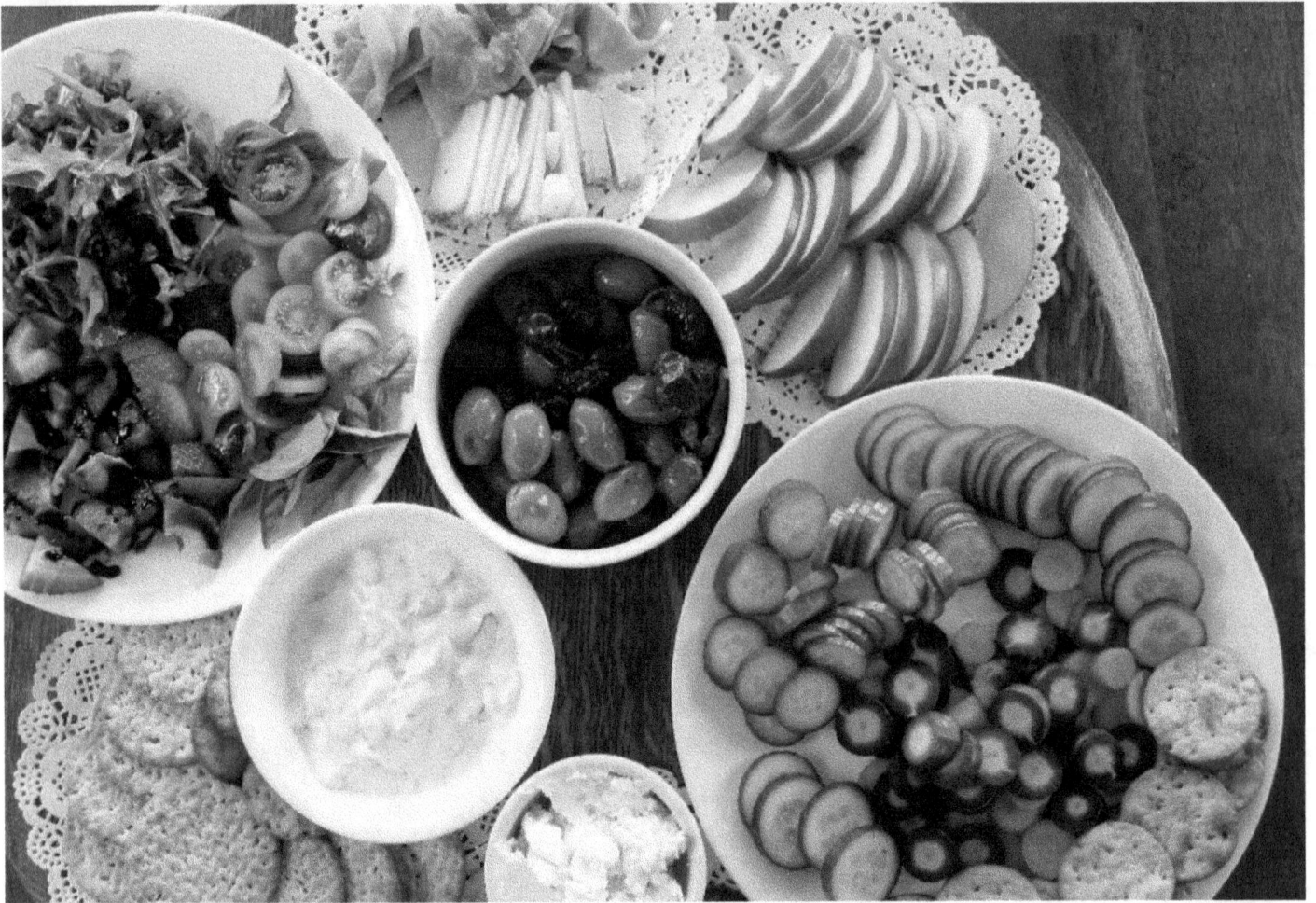

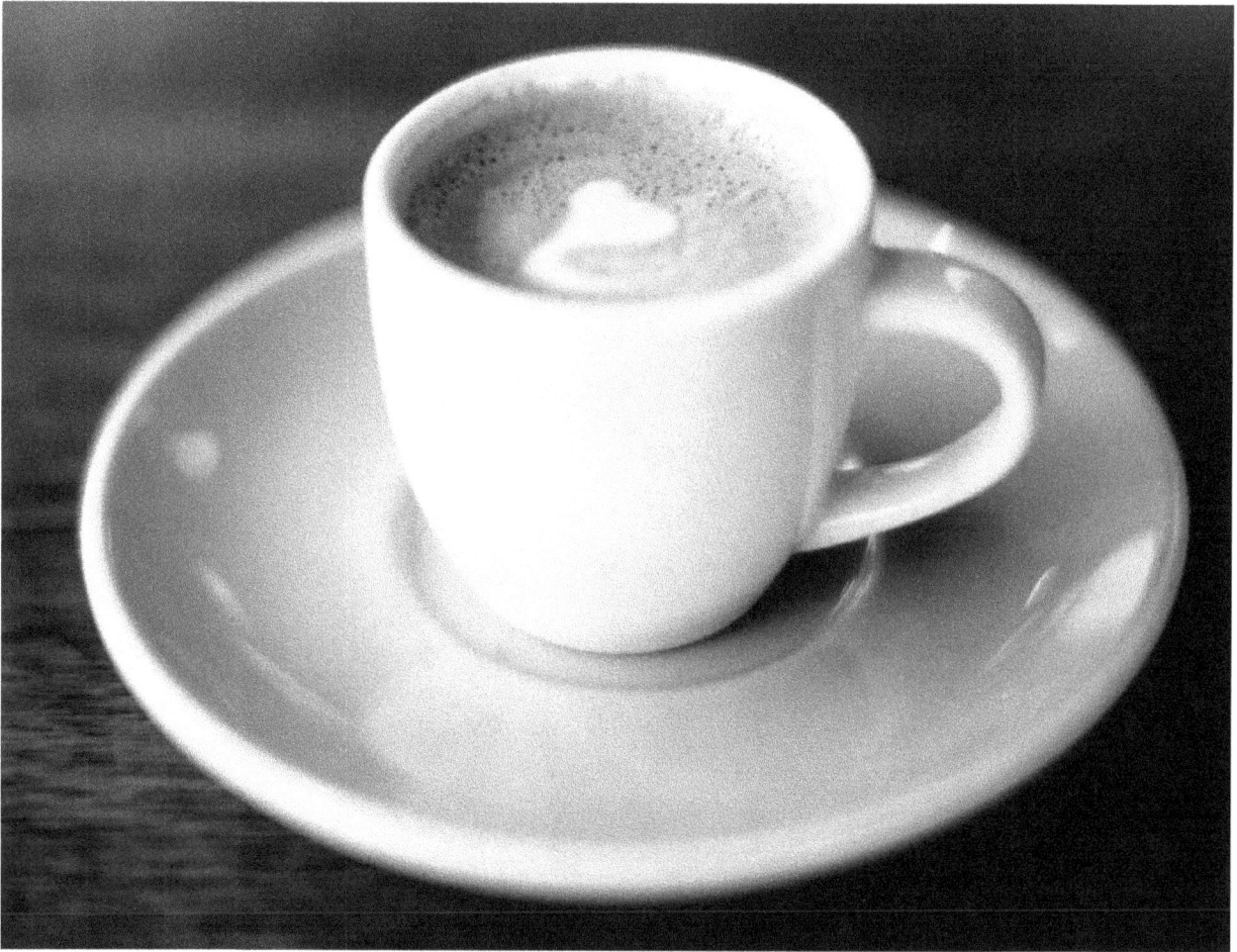

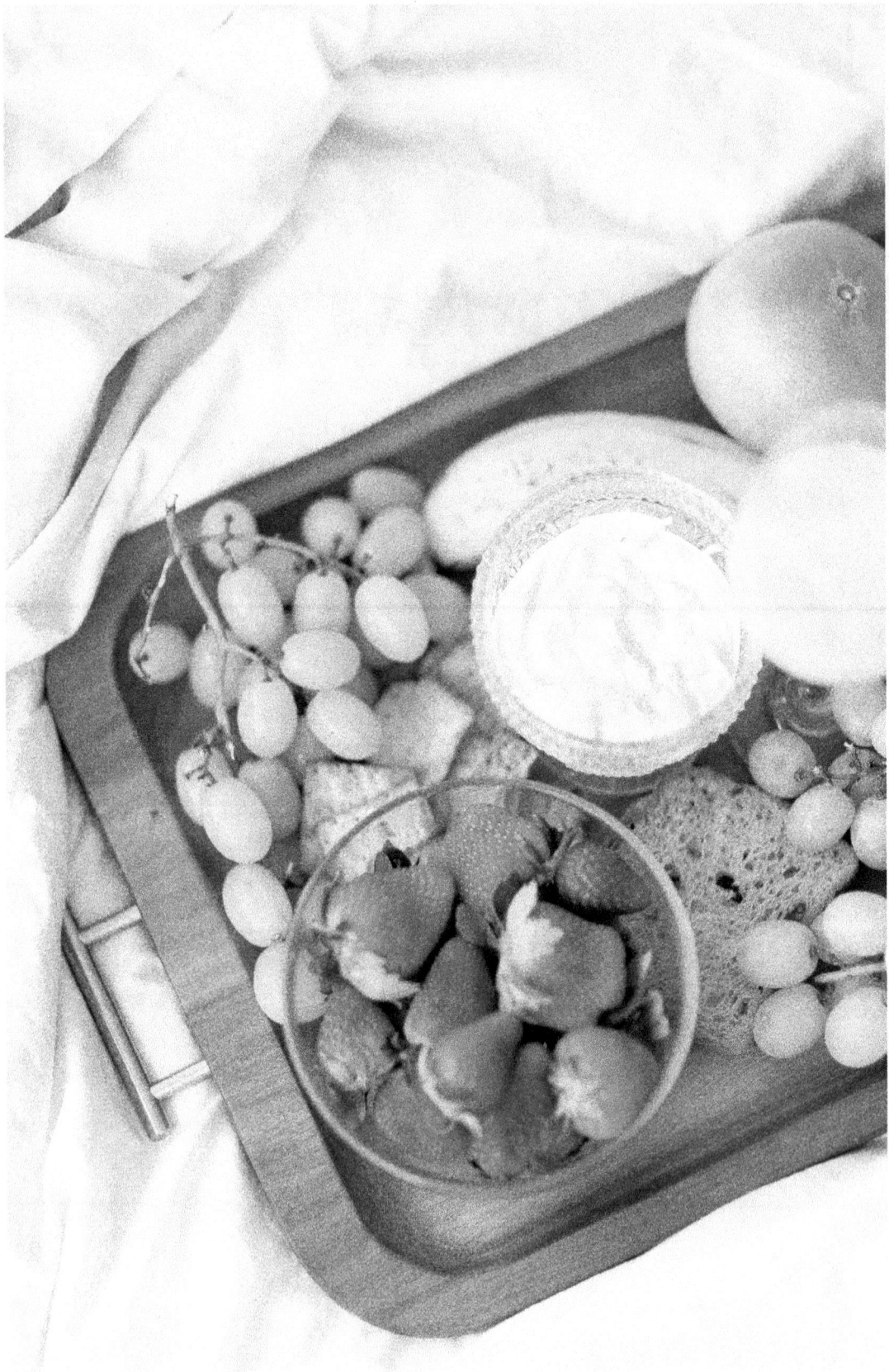

CHAPTER 1:
WHAT IS THE KETOGENIC DIET?

Possibly when we hear about the word diet, the erroneous idea of restricting the free consumption of food and limiting ourselves to only a few nutrients and energies which are considered "necessary" in order to lose weight comes to mind.

Before going into the subject of what could be the ketogenic diet, let's define some concepts, which will be very helpful and supportive for the following chapters.

What does the word Diet mean? This word whose meaning is "regime of life" comes from the Greek word "dayta," this refers to the consumption of food that we do in our day to day (each one with a lapse of 24 hours) to our organism.

With the passing of the years the word diet has acquired much power and importance in the daily life of the human being, whether by leading a good lifestyle, a belief or simply curiosity; currently there are millions of characteristics associated with this word (this could be: low sodium diet, vegetarian diet, reduction diet, keto diet) the important thing is that you must always meet the following characteristics so that it can be called this way, a "diet":

It must be complete; a properly balanced diet must include all the nutrients necessary to provide all those vitamins and minerals that our body needs.

A diet should not imply a risk to our health, just as there are abundant foods in nutrients, there are foods that contain toxins and pollutants for our body, and these must be consumed with much moderation.

At the moment of ingesting the food, our plate must be proportionally balanced (there should not be more nutrients than others, it is suggested that all are the same).

The plate of our food to ingest must cover the sufficient nutrients that we need to have a correct weight. (and in the case of children, good growth and correct development.) It is never advisable to overload our dishes with nutrients to be completely full because being satisfied helps our body a lot.

A correct diet must be varied; it is advisable to include different types of nutrients in each group or portion.

And finally the most important because, to be able to eat well, we have to feel comfortable, our food must be according to our personal taste, this can also influence our culture, economic resources or any other factor.

It is very important to keep in mind that each diet is personalized because each person does not have the same physical condition, depending on this will reflect their mood, physical energy, mental capacity, body humor, physical aspects such as skin, hair, body odors and even health.

Up to this point, we must surely be asking ourselves, How can I start a correct diet if I have led a disordered lifestyle (in terms of my diet)?

To be able to "start" or just eat properly, we must be strong and put aside those treats, reduce certain foods that harm us; these could be: heavy flours, certain cereals, sugary foods, and many other foods that we are used to eating. And the most important thing: it is not to eat less, it is to increase the number of meals per day diminishing the portions in each plate; in this way, we are balancing our organism.

One way to clearly see the example of what a diet is is the ketogenic diet, which is well known for being a low-carbohydrate diet, which helps us burn fat more effectively.

By ingesting carbohydrates, our body produces substances such as glucose and insulin, which our body needs in order to produce energy. Both substances work together within our bloodstream.

MEANING OF KETO

The ketogenic diet was developed at the beginning of the 20th century by doctors, who were looking for a diet based on high-fat consumption, in order to control seizures in children. It had long been observed that fasting worked as a kind of treatment for epilepsy but of course, it was not possible for a person to fast for the rest of his life, which is why they began to use this type of food in epileptic patients where their diet was going to be based on the highest consumption of fat.

Over time it was observed that these patients who had followed the ketogenic style of feeding had decreased their seizures and even in a minority had disappeared seizure attacks.

With these results, certain studies indicated that this type of feeding generated molecules called ketones, which were the reason for the success in reducing epileptic seizures; on the other hand, other studies showed that the shortage of glucose is the reason why these seizures were lightened.

Since this diet is low in carbohydrates and abundant in fats, it allows our body to produce molecules (which we could consider a type of fuel) called "ketones." The ketone would be like a kind of alternative fuel, which our body uses when we have glucose (sugar) deficiency in the blood.

This molecule is produced by the liver by decreasing the intake of carbohydrates and proteins, as they become sugar when absorbed into our bloodstream. As we saw before, ketone becomes a kind of fuel for our body in general, but especially produces a large amount of fuel for our brain. As we know, the brain is considered a kind of computer in our body, this is responsible for processing all kinds of information such as movements, gestures, every word we say or think in our day to day, which is why this organ needs more energy consumption, which in this case would be ketone or glucose.

When we apply the ketogenic diet, our body changes the way we supply that "fuel" to work mainly with the fat we produce. This is burned constantly 24 hours a day, every day of the week. This happens when our insulin levels drop because our body is given access to that fat stored in the body to be burned.

The ketogenic diet is ideal if you need to lose weight as it provides a lot of benefits such as improved concentration, improved energy supply, and something very obvious, feeling more satisfied with each meal.

When we eat this type of diet, our body enters a metabolic state called ketosis, which is nothing more than a natural state in which our body feeds itself entirely on fat.

There are some restrictions on this type of diet. Definitively we can say that the ketogenic diet possesses a great number of benefits. However, this also possesses a certain quantity of "negative" effects, which indicate that their practice could come to be considered dangerous for some people since it influences as much in physical health as their mental health.

To correctly follow the ketogenic diet we must take into account that we will make certain changes in our lifestyle, and therefore we must be prepared physically and mentally for it, this is why it is not recommended to start with this type of food to those people who still consider the excessive consumption of carbohydrates as a fundamental part of their diet, people seeking a temporary solution to lose weight, people who do not maintain a constant routine (as we saw earlier when practicing this diet, our body enters a state of ketosis, and our body needs to be able to adapt to the changes).

In particular, this type of diet is not recommended to all those people who are taking medication or have a special health condition, pregnant women or mothers who are breastfeeding.

WHO SHOULD FOLLOW THIS DIET?

This diet is mostly recommended for all epileptic patients, although most young people find it difficult to follow this type of diet, due to the fact that it requires strict compliance with the way of eating.

Among the possible side effects of this diet are growth retardation (when this diet is applied to children), kidney problems, weight loss, bone weakness, etc.

When a person with an epileptic condition is willing to follow this diet, he or she must spend a few days in the hospital in order to monitor the possible effects to which his or her body may react. Once this has happened, you should have constant control with a nutritionist who can guide the patient on how to serve their portions of food.

PEOPLE WITH TYPE 1 DIABETES

We know that this type 1 diabetes is an autoimmune disease, where the immune system attacks the pancreas, destroying the cells that detect sugar in the blood and are responsible for creating insulin; when this happens, the body is unable to absorb glucose, and the accumulated sugar could increase in a very dangerous way.

Therefore, patients with type 1 diabetes must maintain constant monitoring of their blood sugar levels; in addition, they must inject certain amounts of insulin to regulate this. This disease is very common in adults over 30 years old, although there are cases of people whose disease was detected in childhood.

People who suffer from this can present complications in their organism, such as hypertension, eye damage, damage to the nervous system, damage to the renal system, and can even develop heart disease. It is for this reason that the ketogenic diet can greatly influence its improvement since by lowering blood sugar, the need for insulin would be reduced by up to 70%; clearly, this must always be with absolutely strict obedience to the ketogenic diet.

It is very important to stick to this diet because if you fail or cheat with some food, you could put your body in a dangerous and deadly state known as ketoacidosis; this happens when ketone molecules accumulate in the blood, reacting in an aggressive way and making this blood become acidic.

PEOPLE WITH TYPE 2 DIABETES

This type of diabetes is the result of a bad nutritional lifestyle in which sugar levels are elevated to very high levels, thus creating insulin resistance, this is nothing more than an inability on the part of the body to make use of the hormone that produces insulin.

It could be very contradictory to apply the ketogenic diet to type 2 diabetic patients, as most of these are patients with obesity, and adding a diet high in fat would be somewhat confusing. But this could be seen as a misunderstanding in the information of carbohydrates and calories as they are not all the same.

Calories, unlike carbohydrates, are capable of reducing appetite, causing a type 2 diabetic to reduce his or her calorie intake. Additionally, it also decreases the production of ghrelin; this is informally known as the hormone that produces appetite, and it also increases the production of amylin and leptin; informally known as the hormones that make us feel satisfied as a result of ketosis.

Type 2 diabetes patients are also very susceptible to ketoacidosis, so it is very important that they are in constant medical checkups and maintain a balanced diet provided by a nutritionist.

CHAPTER 2: KETO MYTHS

Because this type of diet may look a little strict or a lot, depending on your point of view, many myths arise about the keto diet. Like the following:

- When you enter ketosis, your body goes towards ketoacidosis: What does this mean? For as you already know, ketosis means that blood sugar levels are low, so the body goes into ketosis, turning fat into energy; if that's the case, you can start losing fat and so on, but now ketoacidosis is something absolutely different, because this is a medical condition, which is extremely serious, because it is produced by low levels of insulin, and very, very high levels of ketones, which could become fatal, we can say that this condition is found in some diabetic patients. Seeing both concepts, we can observe that they are diametrically different things, since one is a healthy condition of the body, which allows the burning of fats in a natural way, and the other is a clinical condition of patients with diabetes.

- The keto diet is based only on the elimination of carbohydrates: This is completely false, since the basis of the keto diet is not only that but is also based on a very high consumption of fats, in addition, it does not seek to eliminate by complete carbohydrates, but requires an efficient consumption of them, the minimum really, but does not prohibit the consumption of them, since it is based on a set of conditions that must be met to get to ketosis, which involves obtaining energy through fat and not sugars that provide us with carbohydrates.

- Muscle is lost while doing the ketogenic diet: This is false, because the keto, is extremely used for athletes, but this myth arises from a confusion, because there is a process in the body, which converts protein into glucose, and as you know, our body is not able to break down fat into glucose. For this reason people think that muscle would be lost, but they can not be further from reality, since almost nothing is converted into glucose, for this reason, it is understood that you get to the false conclusion that you lose muscle, but for the muscles to be maintained, or grow, it is something absolutely amazing, because to get started, the muscles necessarily use glucose, therefore, there are processes in our body that are dependent on glucose, but there are others that are not, and the same tasks that some organs can perform with glucose, they can perform with ketones, one of these organs capable of doing this is the brain, the amazing process that the human body is the following, the little glucose that the body generates goes to the brain, but in this case, the brain depends on ketones, and a certain amount of them will go to the brain, and the glucose that was intended for that organ, will go to the muscles, so as to maintain muscle mass or increase the size of them.

- All people need the same amounts of carbohydrates: This is totally false since not everyone has the same needs because they depend on the individual health conditions of each person. Therefore, it is likely that some people will not be able to make a strict ketogenic diet right away, as they may be affected by such a drastic change in their dietary intake, this may also depend on their daily physical activity.

- The ketogenic diet limits the consumption of certain foods: This is absolutely true, as many of the foods it restricts are cereals, sweets, sugary drinks, processed foods and lots of fruits, as most of its composition is based on carbohydrates, thus becoming, into fructose in the body and making the process of ketosis more difficult, and that energy would not be produced thanks to fats and ketones, but to sugars in our body.

- The ketogenic diet slows down your metabolism: This is because when people hear the word diet, comes to mind the slowing of the metabolism, and this is because, in the vast majority of diets, a large decrease in calorie consumption, in the long run, will generate a slowing of the metabolism of people who make such diets. In order to avoid this and make use of ketosis, it is good that one day, we proceed to eat carbohydrates, of course not in a big excess, but you will skip the diet, so to speak. After that, you can resume ketosis, because there will come a time when you can reach the state of ketosis very quickly. But it is that really, this diet has something very particular, since this allows to maintain the same metabolism or could even increase it, since it makes a high consumption of calories, and allows you to lose weight, thus achieving to be a diet that carries out something totally different to the other diets, because the common ones are characterized by a low caloric consumption and these are able to slow down the metabolism. Although we already mentioned that the ketogenic diet does not slow down the metabolism, it is not a bad practice, as previously said, to consume sometimes a greater amount of carbohydrates.

- Eating so many fats is harmful to health: This is a myth, since there are good fats and bad fats, which are harmful are those found in frying oils, butter and trans fats, but there are also good fats, those found in food without the need to go through chemical processes, such as avocados, coconut oil, among others, as there are many people who believe they have to eat fried foods, butter, hamburgers, pizzas, because the ketogenic diet is based on the consumption of fats, but on the good consumption of them. Good fats are vital to the body for various reasons, among which are found to be responsible for the constitution of cell membranes, transport fat-soluble vitamins, and as if this were not enough, also provides energy to the body. Therefore, we can say that the human body needs fats for its proper functioning, but in a good proportion.

- Ketogenic diets are high in protein: This is false for several reasons, the first is that a high intake of protein is going to become fructose or sugar in our blood so to speak, which causes it to leave the state of ketosis, therefore, affects the purpose of the diet, which is to get to be at that level to burn fat, another point that affects the high intake of protein, is that the decomposition of amino acids that are obtained in proteins, produce an increase in the number of ketones found in our body, but although this sounds attractive for the purposes of the keto diet, the same is hazardous to health, since a disproportionate amount of ketones in our body more than a benefit can become a risk.

- The ketogenic diet involves not eating for long periods of time: This is false, since this type of diet never requires long periods of time without eating, but rather a low-carbohydrate diet, which is the basis of the keto diet, but although there is no restriction when consuming food, it is also true that fasting is very useful and beneficial to lose weight, but the fundamental principle of keto, is to make a complete food plan, which allows people to nourish themselves and feel satiated when eating, consuming quality fat, thus producing high levels of energy that do not depend on the fructose generated by carbohydrates, but fat, thanks to ketones

- The ketogenic diet does not allow to consume sweets or desserts: This is false, since the keto, is based on not consuming carbohydrates or processed foods such as sugars, but there are desserts that do not have anything of that in their preparation, such as those based on nuts, Greek yogurt, chocolate, in addition, that these are sweetened with natural sweeteners such as stevia, because as you know, it does not have fructose. Therefore, we can get sweets such as cheesecakes, brownies, or even biscuits, and there is no need for any of the traditional ingredients that would take us out of the state of ketosis. These recipes will be explained later, as the book progresses.

These are some of the myths that we can get with the ketogenic diet, as you can see, there are still people who do not believe in it by this type of myth, it will only depend on you whether to believe in the keto or not.

CHAPTER 3:
BENEFITS OF USING KETO

When we talk about ketogenic feeding we can think that the only benefit or the one that stands out, at first sight, is the considerable weight loss, which is in fact achieved quickly, but not only is the weight loss the benefit that is achieved with this diet, as we have commented previously, in its beginnings this diet was applied in adults and children who suffered from epileptic seizures.

Improvements have also been observed in people suffering from convulsions and problems in their cognitive functions.

It has also been noted that in people who have certain brain conditions, the keto diet has some curative properties when done, such as neurodegenerative diseases, epilepsy. In addition to being able to raise endorphin levels, thus raising moods, as well as improvements in concentration, raises melatonin levels, helping to better sleep and regulate our circadian cycle.

In addition, this diet considerably lowers blood sugar levels, which is why it is widely recommended for diabetics. This is mainly due to the fact that by decreasing carbohydrate consumption, we are going to decrease blood sugar levels. When we eat carbohydrates, these foods are digested and transformed into glucose in the blood, in that sense starts to act insulin which is the hormone that is responsible for sending all that glucose to cells to consume it or in its absence and that is actually what always happens, to be stored. There are cases in which the cells stop responding to insulin, and in this way, the control of glucose in the blood is lost, and this is when we have a serious problem because we would be talking about suffering from type 2 diabetes. But in patients who have been treated with this ketogenic diet and exercise, considerable improvements have been found. In fact, many of the people have considerably decreased the consumption of their medications since applying it.

Cardiovascular improvements are also obtained, thus improving all the indicators that determine the risk of suffering cardiovascular diseases, it has been shown in various studies that although this diet increases fat consumption, cholesterol levels improve, this means that there is a higher percentage of good cholesterol HDL and LDL-C, there is also a large decrease in triglyceride levels and improvements in blood pressure of people who practice it. Against all odds when some critics thought that this type of food could alter cholesterol levels and triglycerides, as it has been determined that the opposite happens.

Taking the body to the state of ketosis one of the most noticeable changes is the decrease in body fat and less visceral fat, the subcutaneous fat is the fat that we can feel or in its defect pinch and that we can get in our arms, legs, belly and other places. While visceral fat is that it accumulates around the organs and that could, in some cases, cause us or increase health risks. With this feeding method, we are able to reduce these two types of fat. Especially there is a considerable decrease in fat in the abdominal cavity.

Ketogenic diets have been used for many years to treat epilepsy problems, but this type of diet is also being studied for diseases such as Alzheimer's, Parkinson's, and this is because ketogenic bodies have neuroprotective effects.

And is that one of the benefits of the keto diet, it has the possibility to feed and heal the brain, this diet is the main source of energy of the brain.

The digestive system is considered as the second brain we have, the intestine has a structure like a mesh, and this mesh is pierced or perforated by anti-nutrients and gluten, which is what is known in medicine as a permeable intestine, this pathology achieves an inflammatory process in the body that is able to improve with the keto, this diet is able to help regulate the digestive system.

Dopamine is a molecule produced in a natural way by our organism, within its functions we have the pleasure, learning, decision making, coordination of movements, motivation, and when we are in the presence of dopamine the reward systems of our brain are going to activate and in this way respond the stimulus that has a positive charge in each one of us. Dopamine helps in the process of remembering some information. Now the low levels of dopamine are directly related to states of depression, attention deficit disorders, hyperactivity, Parkinson's, hyperthyroidism. But the good news is that the keto diet increases dopamine levels, so it's advisable to eat this way.

When we reach the level of ketosis, there are many advantages and benefits that we acquire with this. There is a decrease in inflammation at a general level in the body, decreases oxidative stress, being these neuroprotective, antitumor. It increases our immune system, so we can conclude that another benefit is to improve autoimmune diseases.

With all that we have mentioned previously we cannot consider the ketogenic diet only to lose weight, we already know that it is a diet that metabolizes fat in an effective and efficient way, if we have an excess of fat our body will use it, otherwise it will use the fat you eat as a fuel and when it needs more fuel will let you know through hunger.

Reaching these ketogenic levels enhances the physical and mental performance of each one of those who practice it, and this is because, in ketosis, blood glucose levels are always stable, so we will not suffer from symptoms of hypoglycemia. We become healthier, and in addition, we do not have any secondary effect, the key is not to fail, is to achieve in principle to detoxify our body of all the antinutrients that are hosted in the body, once achieved this step we will see how easy it is to implement this food plan.

Migraines are classified as a neurological disorder, the lack of energy in neurons is one of the causes of these migraines, it is well known that there are many treatments that have been tried for migraines, but we have good news, ketosis can eliminate this disorder, hypoglycemia is associated with headache, when we are on a normal diet, glucose is the sole fuel for the brain, so the energy we need for neurons is not enough, but this does not happen with ketones, as an alternative fuel. Since ketones are then the most effective fuel for the brain, the heart, and also the intestine, they preserve and promote the creation of muscle mass, promote the generation of new mitochondria, and finally increases longevity in each of the people who practice it.

The ketogenic diet activates the necessary genes to be able to use fat as the main fuel, and sugar as a secondary fuel, so we can say that we are going to have two fuel tanks, one coming from fats where millions of kcal can be stored, and another tank of sugar or glycogen and which is also very limited since it has approximately 2000 kcal. When we use the sugar tank we spend it quickly so we will need to refill this tank and get again the fuel we need, but if on the contrary, we use fat fuel with the keto diet, we will have an inexhaustible tank of fuel and available at any time, could there be a better benefit of it?. The keto diet is a wonderful tool to improve our health.

CHAPTER 4:
KETOSIS AND MENTAL HEALTH

To begin this section, the first thing we need to know or define is, what is health? And what is a better definition than what the world health organization can offer us? It says that literally "Health is a state of complete physical, mental and social well-being, and not only the absence of disease or illness", therefore, we can say that health is not only the lack of physical illnesses, but that one must also be mentally and psychologically balanced, in addition to being socially good with others, since many studies have shown that a person who is not psychologically well will not have physical health either. Moreover, cancer patients often make psychological therapies so that they can recover faster since emotionally stable patients have a higher percentage of recovery.

Therefore, we recommend that you first try to be mentally stable because no matter how much ketogenic diet you do, you will not be able to have a complete integral health, therefore it is always good to have the three stable states of health, both physical, emotional and social.

After having mentioned the importance of the integral health, we can explain the importance of the ketogenic diet to be able to improve our physical health, since this not only helps us to reduce, since many times, this is the end that is sought to the diets, but the same one has a number of utilities in the scope of the health as you will be able to see next.

Ketosis and Cancer: The keto diet is very useful for cancer patients, because a large part of cancer cells feed on glucose cells and as you should already know that glucose in our body is produced thanks to carbohydrate intake, therefore by drastically lowering their consumption, fewer glucose cells will be created, and the cancer cells will not be able to feed, or not most of them, since almost none of these cells can feed on ketones, so we can stop or slow down the growth rate of the cancer.

Ketosis and diabetes: As you should know, diabetes is a disease that occurs when there is an excessive concentration of glucose in the blood, either because the pancreas does not make enough insulin, and this generates that glucose is not transformed into energy efficiently. Therefore, after knowing this, we can make use of the keto diet, and thus achieve control of glucose in our blood, because we will generate more ketones in our body, and these will do the work of glucose in our body, generating energy through them, thus achieving a better quality of life for patients.

But now, going to the point, ketosis has a great impact on our brain health since first, much of the vital processes for our body is done by the brain with the help of ketosis, but these functions can also be used with the help of ketones. Therefore, we can say that the brain can use the cells that are produced when practicing the ketogenic diet to perform their vital functions.

One of the first benefits we can see from the ketogenic diet is that it improves the condition of patients suffering from epilepsy, which is a brain disorder that occurs when there is electrical overactivity in some specific areas of the brain, people who suffer from this, may suffer convulsions or unwanted movements, when these seizures occur are called epileptic seizures. But then, for a treatment, or help that can be done to patients suffering from epilepsy, is the use of the ketogenic diet, since the diet is able to reduce to a very high degree the frequency of seizures that can occur to patients suffering from epilepsy, of course this does not mean that patients should stop taking their pills to control the disease, but the keto diet could be a great help in reducing the frequency of seizures, because as you know, the ketogenic diet makes a high increase in the level of ketones in the blood, thus making a better control of seizures.

Most of the time this diet is prescribed, it is scoped for children, and the statistical results of patients with epilepsy, we can find that there are cases that range between 10% and 15% who do not suffer from seizures again, there are also other cases in which more than 50% of patients who are instructed to follow the diet, the frequency in which seizures occur is reduced to at least half the time. How does the ketogenic diet help patients with seizures? Well, since we have a high level of ketosis, it allows us to alter the genes that are related to the brain's energetic metabolism, since the brain will take ketones as its main source of nutrition, instead of glucose, which implies that neuronal functions will be controlled, which are those that are affected at the time of the seizures. Also to verify the result of the keto diet in our brain, regarding that disease, we can observe that there was a substantial increase in the energy reserves of the neurons of the hippocampus, increasing the number of mitochondria, therefore, increasing the concentration of mitochondria in the hippocampus, meaning that the density of mitochondria in the hippocampus increased a lot, this means that energy production in the hippocampus is improved, which may mean that better neuronal stability will be obtained.

On the other hand there are other brain diseases that can be improved through the practice of the ketogenic diet, such as Alzheimer, which is a brain disease, better said is a progressive cognitive disorder that will degenerate brain cells, which leads to problems of memory, thinking, and behavior, such disease is gradually worsening, leading to the death of people suffering from that disease. There is no way to end the disease, there are only treatments to slow its degenerative process, but there is no way to eliminate it. But in order for these patients to achieve a better quality of life, the ketogenic diet can be recommended, since the ketones in the brain could reactivate some neurons, thus repairing part of the brain damage caused by Alzheimer's, since thanks to the help of ketones, we can try to prolong the life of these neurons, also taking care of our dendrites and axons, thus achieving, or better said, trying to achieve better connections in the brain to try to make synapses. This being the main damage of Alzheimer's disease, as it does not allow a good synapse in the brain, thus placing increasingly difficult barriers in patients to use their brain, either to remember things or do daily activities. Although it cannot be said that there is irrefutable evidence that the ketogenic diet can stop Alzheimer's or put an end to it, what we can say is that they have carried out a series of experiments on animals, which already have brain degeneration, something very similar to those suffered by these types of patients, and it can be said that the animals that were on a ketogenic diet, could perform the tasks in a better way to the animals that were not on it; on the other hand, studies were made on mice in their juvenile stage, which had brain lesions, and it could be observed that those to whom the ketogenic diet was applied, the brain was protected from damage, but not only that, there were cases in which it was possible to regenerate brain damage. Therefore, we can say that the ketogenic diet could be hopeful for those patients suffering from Alzheimer's disease.

These are some of the diseases with which the ketogenic diet can help us, but there are also others that would be just as useful to have a better quality of life, to mention some other brain disease that this diet could help brain cancer could be one of them, by this we do not mean that the diseases are eliminated only by making the diet, because it is not magic either, but we can say that it could improve the quality of life of the patient, and it is also very good for the patient to be in better condition to take the treatment with his doctor of confidence.

CHAPTER 5:

KETOGENIC NUTRITION

When starting a ketogenic diet, we must take into account very important factors such as our dietary habits; the amount of food we eat each day with its consistency (this includes heavy or light meals).

In addition, we must take into account important factors of our body, such as our body weight and height, consider if we are consuming any pharmacological treatment, perform previous blood tests to discard any weakness that may occur in our body.

The ketogenic diet has an innumerable variety of benefits, we have already seen how it can improve brain functions, helps hormonal regulation in women, has been used for patients suffering from epileptic seizures, and so an endless list of benefits that has managed to place this diet as one of the most requested and as one of the most researched.

But it has also arisen the need to know if this method of feeding possesses nutrients of high value for our organism, and is that although the main restriction of the keto diet is the elimination of the carbohydrates and of the refined sugars and flours, the foods that are allowed are of high nutritional content.

If we learn to know our body and the nutritional contents of food, we can make a significant change in our lives. One of the food groups that is consumed most in this diet is vegetables. It is recommended to consume many green foods, such as spinach, celery, or celery, Spain, parsley, all with high nutritional properties and large amounts of magnesium.

Another of the foods that are used in this plan is the consumption of meat, chicken, pork or fish, although in other diets this type of food is restricted, this is a diet that prioritizes the consumption of natural and healthy fats, without affecting cholesterol levels or triglyceride levels, whitefish are lean options that are both reduced calories, fish is a high-quality protein and a wonderful source of omega 3, which provides innumerable benefits for the health of our body, the main idea of ketogenic food is to reduce as much as possible the consumption of carbohydrates to be able to produce ketone bodies or ketosis.

Olive oil is a key element and nutritious, is an excellent source of quality fat for the body, olive oil has antioxidant and anti-inflammatory properties. It is also a high-quality oil, but it is always advisable to use it in a moderate way and avoid fried foods when preparing meals.

The avocado is a fruit widely used in this diet, is a vegetable protein that provides antioxidant benefits as well as vitamins and minerals, the avocado is rich in potassium, in addition to having fatty acids that are very beneficial for cardiovascular health, have a large amount of fiber, help lower cholesterol levels and triglycerides. It is a food that you can use to prepare breakfast, lunch, or dinner, and as you can see, the food is also focused on improving your health.

The egg is also an allowed food and provides us fat and protein, vitamin B1, A, D, B2, and niacin, with which we can make a lot of dishes, and complements for other meals.

Nuts and seeds are also recommended in this diet, rich in fiber and natural fats, omega3, antioxidants, in addition to seeds and nuts can make a large number of dishes, whether keto bread, tortillas, butter, and even chocolate creams, because as you acquire more knowledge on the subject and the properties of the food you are consuming, you can be able to prepare dishes or highly nutritious menus and with the goal of finally reaching nutritional ketosis.

Fresh cheeses are rich in protein with a low amount of saturated fat and sodium, are a rich source of calcium, vitamin A and D. There are also vegan cheeses that, in addition to being very rich, there is a wide variety of them.

in the ketogenic diet there are different types within it, there is the classic ketogenic diet rich in fat, where about 90% of the diet consumed is fat, this diet is adjusted to the energy amounts of each individual, in general, it is managed in the following way: for every 3 or 4 grams of fat consumed, a gram of protein is offered together. however, this is not always the case, depending on the needs of each person, the diet will be adjusted depending on its ketogenic capacity.

There is also the ketogenic diet with medium-chain triglycerides MCT diet proposed in 1971 by Huttenlocher. In this diet, the type of fat is consumed as MCT oil, and it is that MCT lipids are metabolized faster than long-chain triglycerides LCT, and thus allow ketosis more quickly.

WHAT STEPS SHOULD BE FOLLOWED FOR THE PROPER FUNCTION OF THIS DIET?

As the ketogenic diet is a complex level diet, it is very important that each step is strictly followed without any mistakes.

It does not matter if we make this diet by our own decision or to improve our health and physical condition or if we suffer from some type of disease (such as epilepsy, diabetes among others) which would benefit us in health, it is very important to go to a nutritionist to give us the necessary guidance not to harm our health and to inform us correctly how to follow the ketogenic diet.

In the case of children, it is very important that they comply with all the rules of the balanced diet without any failure; since, as they are in a growth stage, these changes will mark a great change in their organism and cognitive development. As we already know, each diet is personal, and for this reason, not all diets are appropriate for all children (regardless of whether they are the same age, weight or size).

Nutritionists usually mainly evaluate the number of nutrients consumed in the first three days of starting this new style of nutrition in order to observe in detail how our body reacts to the changes and even in some cases, supervises a disease.

TYPES OF KETOGENIC DIET

There are different types of cytogenetic diet, and that is why we must be very attentive to which is the most appropriate according to our physical and mental condition.

CYCLIC CYTOGENETIC DIET

This type of diet is one in which, as its name says, a cycle is going to be followed in which a plan of certain periods for consuming carbohydrates is included, for example: 6 days of strict compliance with the ketogenic diet and one day of carbohydrates.

STANDARD KETOGENIC DIET

This is the type of diet where your low-carbohydrate meal plan moderates carbohydrate intake and most foods will be fat-based. This will normally range from 75% to 80% fat, 15% to 20% protein and only 5% or less carbohydrate intake.

HIGH PROTEIN KETOGENIC DIET

This type of diet is one in which food distribution is as follows: 60% fat, 5% carbohydrate, and 35% protein. In other words, this diet will be performing the functions of the standard cytogenetic diet but will add more protein than usual.

It is important to note that these percentages may vary according to the needs of our body and condition.

ADAPTED CYTOGENETIC DIET

This is the type of diet in which we are allowed to consume carbohydrates on the days we exercise.

Mostly, cyclic or adapted diets are used for more professional purposes by health experts, athletes or bodybuilders as they have a deeper knowledge of their body and are able to handle any type of situation with their body.

CHAPTER 6:
INTERMITTENT FASTING

Increasingly more people are interested in practicing intermittent fasting, as every day are more known the broad benefits that can be achieved by our body to apply it. Today, the word "intermittent fasting" has practically become a worldwide trend, particularly in the field of fitness and methods to lose weight more quickly and without rebound effect, which is what mainly concerns people who make different diets.

Intermittent fasting is a physiological mechanism that has been practiced since our ancestors, fasting is absolutely beneficial to health, and is something that has been practiced throughout history.

But which are the results that we can obtain when applying the intermittent fast, that encourages us to apply it, well, the intermittent fast regulates the glucose in blood, improves the arterial pressure, improves the focus and mental clarity, helps notably in the process of detoxification, increases considerably the levels of energy of our body, increases the productivity of different hormones in our organism, like the growth hormone, reduces the rate of aging, prevents the cancer, cellular regeneration, among many of the other benefits.

Intermittent fasting is very important and consists of not eating food for an estimated time. Fasting daily between 16-22 hours is a health tool that decreases the risk of disease.

When we do the intermittent fasting insulin levels go down when these levels go down, the body draws energy from the liver and fats, and when we fast continuously our body will achieve a good balance and begins the keto-adaptation. Intermittent fasting works because when we lower insulin levels, the body begins to burn fat.

The best way to go with intermittent fasting is with the ketogenic diet, exercise. Intermittent fasting allows the hormones to do their job correctly, during this period of time that we do not ingest any food there is no insulin, and in its absence, counter-regulating hormones such as growth hormone, glucagon, adrenaline, etc., can initiate pathways for cell repair and thus clean our body of metabolic waste, helping the growth of muscle mass, to access our body fat that begins to be intelligently used by our body as energy, begins the production of ketones in the liver and increases basal caloric expenditure.

When we fast intermittently, increases the production of growth hormones (GH), as mentioned above, but what does this hormone do in our body? does three fundamental things: it favors lipolysis, increasing the oxidation of fats, thus helping the production of ketones, also helps maintain muscle mass inhibiting muscle degradation to make glucose, and finally prevents us from presenting symptoms of hypoglycemia.

We have to understand that when we eat and when we suppress ourselves from food we generate hormones that have different mechanisms of action, for example, when we practice fasting, meaning that we do not eat for certain periods of time, we generate more growth hormones, adrenaline or glucagon, while when we feed, we generate insulin hormone. At present, people are suffering from hyperinsulinemia and growth hormone deficiency, which leads us to conclude that it is necessary and advisable to apply intermittent fasting accompanied by ketogenic feeding.

There are currently various modalities of intermittent fasting, but we will mention the three most important, remember that it is not a rule to apply and that everyone can apply it according to their own requirements and the recommendations of the specialist. The categories of intermittent fasting that we have summarized among so many types of fasting that there are are are the following:

INTERMITTENT FASTING (IF)

This voluntary fast restricts the intake of solid food for a period of time between 16-48 hours. You can also restrict the consumption of food for a period of time of 6-8 hours.

PERIODIC FASTING (PF)

Buchinger type fast. Büchinger's fasting method consists of a limited intake of fruit juices as well as small amounts of vegetable broth being the nutritional energy consumption of 200 to 400 kcal/day. Exercise is also practiced with this method, mind-body techniques, the application of enemas and the taking of laxative salts.

INTERMEDIATE 24/7 FASTING

This type of intermittent fasting consists of having only 4 hours a day to eat, thus leaving the other 20 hours of fasting; this could be summed up as two meals and even one per day.

This type of fast could offer very promising results because, as we have seen, it is very difficult to be surpassed with food feeding us at most twice a day.

Now, the implementation of any of these types of fasting carries with it a series of results that have been cataloged as beneficial:

On the circadian rhythm, a study with overweight individuals ate for only 10-11 hours a day for 16 weeks and not only they were able to reduce body weight, burn localized fat and manifest to be full of energy, in addition, there were improvements in sleep, and the benefits persisted for one year.

The most common eating pattern in society today is to eat three meals a day plus snacks, in animal and human studies suggest that intermittent fasting, when the fasting period is extended to 16 hours, can improve health indicators and thus counteract disease processes. Changes in fat metabolism occur, and ketones are produced, as well as stimulation of adaptive cellular stress responses that prevent and also repair molecular damage.

Improvements in the antitumor effect have been observed, improving the mechanisms of autophagy, due to these studies Yoshinori Ohsumi has been awarded the Nobel Prize in 2016

Intermittent fasting and fasting itself has the potential to delay aging, and especially brain aging, in animal studies, it has been shown that daily caloric restriction, intermittent fasting, and fasting on alternate days, modifies the sensory pathways of nutrients in the brain, increasing synaptic plasticity, neurogenesis, and neuroprotection.

Recent small trials of intermittent fasting in patients with cancer or multiple sclerosis have generated promising results that provide a strong rationale for moving forward with larger clinical trials.

WHAT IS AUTOPHAGY?

Our organism requires periods of maximum intensity and periods of absolute rest, and we can notice this in the bright light we receive during the day, where many chemical, physiological and biological processes occur in our organism, and later we have a period of rest, when night arrives, where certain processes also occur, the same thing happens with temperature changes and the same thing happens with food, the body needs moments or periods of food nutrition but also needs periods of abstinence and regeneration. When we practice intermittent fasting, for example, we give our body those periods it needs.

When we practice intermittent fasting, something called autophagy occurs, and it can be explained in the following way: in 1974, Christian de Duve discovered the lysosomes, and observed that they had the capacity to recycle cellular scrap, that is, dysfunctional mitochondria, bacteria, and even viruses, and converted them into new functional molecules.

In this way, the cell would be feeding on its own damaged parts to renew itself, and hence the term or expression "autophagy." If we did not live this important process of autophagy in the cells, all that cellular scrap would accumulate in our organism causing finally an endless number of diseases and the accelerated aging of the cellular organism.

When we practice fasting, we activate autophagy, and as a consequence of this activation, all the benefits that were mentioned before are achieved. But autophagy does not occur instantaneously by applying intermittent fasting. Rather it is a process that will occur gradually. It is important to emphasize that it is not necessary to do very prolonged fasting in order to reach autophagy; what is important is to be constant with the implementation of intermittent fasting, for example.

You can start implementing 13-hour fasting in the hours of sleep; you can play with different combinations of intermittent fasting:

Elevated frequency: Periods of 12/12 or 16/8, meaning 12 hours of fasting and 12 hours of food intake within the ketogenic diet, or 16 hours of fasting and 8 hours of food intake within the ketogenic diet. This process can be applied several days a week or every day.

Average frequency: Fasting for 24 hours, this type of fast can be done once a week, it should be noted that this kind of practice is recommended to be performed under medical supervision and with prior preparation of our body, it is not recommended under any circumstances to practice without prior information.

Low frequency: fasting or restricting the consumption of solid food for 2-3 days and generally practiced once a month; likewise, this type of practice should be performed under medical supervision.

During fasting, you can consume water, apple vinegar, coffee, water with lemon, tea, but the fat, coconut oil, and green juices do come out of fasting, as carbohydrates and fat stimulate insulin.

How can we break these hours of fasting? Once we spend hours without eating solid food. Autophagy is inhibited by elevations of insulin or the presence of amino acids, but it is very difficult to determine. During fasting is advisable to consume water to which you can add lemon or orange juice, probiotic drinks, bone broth that provides nutrition with the intake of few calories. These are some of the combinations of foods that we recommend to break the fast, since when so many hours go by without ingesting solid foods it is not recommended that when finishing it, one begins ingesting great amounts of food but rather to begin with a tea, a broth of bones, water, and gradually starts ingesting foods within the ketogenic diet.

Fasting is contraindicated for pregnant women, children, anyone who has hormonal alterations, are some of the contraindications that we must take into account before applying the fast, which is why we insist on the fact that before fasting should be consulted with experts because each case is individual.

CHAPTER 7:
BENEFITS OF FASTING

THE ADVANTAGES OF FASTING

One of the most obvious advantages of fasting is weight loss. In ancient times it was called detoxification of the body to all periods of fasting in which the idea was to limit the intake of food for a certain number of hours in order to purify the digestive system. It was believed that if you lasted a while detoxifying, our body will remove all those toxins from it and make us look younger. In a way was right because living a healthy lifestyle, our skin is the first to reflect it.

The correct follow-up of this routine of feeding can offer us a number of benefits to health and even to our physical performance in the day to day. As has been mentioned, the results of these benefits will be those that depend on our willingness to improve eating habits.

This is why when we make a food protocol such as intermittent fasting, we must do it in a proper way because it is useless to fast based on a diet of pre-cooked food, junk, fried and canned or any other food of non-natural origin, since it is going to be the same as continuing to consume these foods in our day to day, every day.

Among the advantages of intermittent fasting that benefits our organism is the following:

- It improves the sensitivity of insulin and glucose as an energy substrate:

As mentioned above, insulin is that hormone produced by the pancreas, which is responsible for capturing glucose as a result of carbohydrate intake (which are stored in the blood to be subsequently released and transported to the point where they will be used to balance glucose levels).

When this hormone becomes so sensitive to our body, there is a higher burning of fat accumulated in our body as a result of the decrease in glycogen within our body in the period of fasting (especially when doing some physical activity). It is for this reason that our body is able to assimilate in a more effective way the glucose that we provide at-home food.

- It helps to lose fat, improve cholesterol, and reduce triglycerides.

As we have mentioned before, one of the main reasons why many people come to this diet looking for a way to burn fat and also improve cholesterol and reduce triglycerides.

Many studies state that physical activity and intermittent fasting can achieve greater fat loss, in turn improving the body system.

- Increases SIRT3, the protein of youth, and reduces mortality.

When our body is in a state of fasting, our body performs a series of processes that favor the growth hormone and youth protein. This hormone makes it difficult for our body to consume glucose, and that is why it is forced to resort to the reserve of accumulated fat in order to obtain energy.

- It helps to reduce the growth of cancer cells.

Fasting is considered a way to reduce the possibility of cancer because when glucose is absent, all those healthy cells automatically begin to burn fat, thus leaving the cancer cells without energy and oxidized to kill them completely.

It also reduces the levels of IGF-1, a hormone linked to insulin, which is considered an engine of cell proliferation considered necessary at the time of physical activity. However, its level can be dangerous when a person has already developed cancer.

- It helps to reduce mortality due to obesity problems.

It has been proven that intermittent fasting can be a good method of disease prevention (which is preventive in the long term). Although it is known that suffering from obesity increases the scope to all types of diseases (heart, glycaemic and many others) which can be deadly, the correct observance of a fast can reduce considerably (or in its entirety) the concentrations of triacylglycerol, the increase in cholesterol and glucose level and can even reduce the possibility of developing diseases such as Alzheimer's disease.

In addition, among the advantages that favor us, the following factors are noteworthy:

- Reduces inflammation.
- It helps us to improve our capacity for self-control in the face of anxiety and lack of food control.
- It has positive effects on the neuronal system.
- It favors autophagy; the organism activates internal recycling mechanisms.

Many investigations have shown that most people prefer to follow an intermittent fasting regime in their long-term eating habits to follow a diet that generates anxiety in terms of food restriction.

These investigations also show that reducing only the intake of calories in their daily diet facilitates much more in the preparation of their food; there have been cases of people who used to consume infinite calories and with only reducing a few have managed to improve their habits without feeling the absence of their dietary change and even achieving a massive loss of weight or excessive fat.

How Does Intermittent Fasting Affect Our Body?

The intermittent fast, in addition to restricting the intake of calories, benefits the hormones of the body to resort to the accumulated fat. In addition, fasting greatly favors the regeneration of those damaged cells of our body.

As for the sensitivity of insulin, it is able to help all (or most) people who suffer from problems of overweight to burn fat more quickly and effectively. Also, while burning fat, at the same time, is generating muscle and that is why these types of diet are more used by bodybuilders and athletes.

Is Intermittent Fasting Recommended for Anyone Who Practices Physical Activity?

As we have been talking about, there is no specific training routine or diet because each person's body assimilates things differently. What we must take into account is that when doing a very intense training (whether cycling, swimming, or running in a marathon) is necessary to consume something that gives us a good performance and, in this case, a fast would not be ideal for these types of situation.

The same could be applied to people who do not perform physical activities of high performance but mild physical activities, but who perform it in high weather conditions of temperature and humidity, as the body will need the consumption of more energy to adapt to the situation in which it is and will not have sufficient nutrients.

It is for this reason that at the moment of carrying out an intermittent fast, it is necessary to take into account the level of demand, conditions to which we are exposed, and duration during our training. In addition, we must always take into account the time that has elapsed since the last meal until the start of training, making sure that we have digested our food correctly.

Surely we have heard that a training in fast is usually much more recommended and we will think that this is a contradiction, a training in fast is always good for the health of the person as long as the duration of this is equal or less than an hour, with a low intensity (or moderately high). In this way, the body adapts slowly to work in low glycogen conditions.

Fasting when exercising is not recommended for all those who have suffered from any type of eating disorder (such as anorexia or bulimia), people with diabetes or hypoglycemia as it can be harmful to your body.

It is very common to think that this method of intermittent fasting is something new that has been used in recent years, while it is true that it has been a method that has gained popularity in recent years, in fact, this method of feeding comes from primitive times because they had no option to access food and had to go out in search of them.

In the same way, it will always be advisable for each person to evaluate what method can result from this protocol, and in this way, observe how it influences their daily workday or exercise. In this way, you are checking what your body needs and if it is able to handle it.

CHAPTER 8:
FASTING FOR WEIGHT LOSS

We already have previous knowledge of what fasting is all about. We know what it means to abstain from eating, drinking or both, for a period of time chosen by the fasting practitioner.

Fasting is a process that has been practiced for many years, from our ancestors and in different cultures, in fact, there are populations that practice fasting and are long-lasting populations, practicing fasting, exercise, and good food. But fasting today is also widely used to lose weight. However, more than a tool to lose weight, it is a lifestyle to improve health, as we have seen in previous cases.

To apply the fast in our organism to lose weight helps to eliminate the accumulated fat of the body and to lose weight, in the same way it helps to take advantage of the energy that is used for the digestion in other processes of the organism, to be able this way to give a rest to some of our organs. The fasting serves to cleanse and detoxify the body. It is always advisable to seek help from specialists before applying fasting because, when applied incorrectly can also have harmful consequences on our body, so it is important not only to investigate but to know our body and be guided by a specialist at the beginning of this very beneficial process.

In order to lose weight, several types of fasting have been implemented:

There are fasts that are applied for a long period, and this fast can last several weeks or even months, depending on the desired results and the physiological conditions of each organism. In this stage, all carbohydrates and calories are eliminated and what is mainly consumed is only liquid. The main objective of this fast is to quickly reach the levels of ketosis in our body. But we must compensate for this lack of food with supplements, minerals guided by specialists, depending exclusively on the conditions and particular requirements of each person.

Juice fasting is a type of fasting in which the main food are fruit juices. There are several fasting protocols like this one that are applied for specific diseases including cancer, a well-known, and applied therapy for healing and detoxification is the "Gerson therapy." In this type of fast, all the necessary nutrients must be incorporated for our bodies. At the same time, it helps the body to improve digestion, and this is achieved in this case by not consuming any solid food.

Alternate fasting is very often used by experts for weight loss and fat burning, in this case, you can get to have a full day without eating food and alternate with normal days where food is consumed in a restricted or controlled way following the ketogenic diet naturally. It is fast, and just like those mentioned above, it must be prescribed by experts. We must have the knowledge not only to follow and stick to them but to get the expected results because if not applied correctly, it can also bring consequences to our health.

Periodic fasting, which differs from intermittent fasting in that this type of fasting is applied for a certain time, but there are more days of normal feeding or where solid foods are allowed, in this case, the fasting can be done on a specific day, could be a specific day a week, for example, and the rest of the week the person has permission to consume the foods permitted within the ketogenic diet.

Intermittent fasting is currently the best known and applied by all or most people who apply the ketogenic diet in which they are going to consume food for a specific period of time, and then spend another period without food or consuming liquids that do not break with the fasting applied, for example, you can fast for 16 hours, managing to stop eating food during that period and after it consuming food within the ketogenic diet, also and following the same steps you can fast for 18 and 20 hours, everything will always depend on your purpose, your preparation, and your body mainly.

Fasting as already mentioned, must be applied with absolute knowledge of what we want to achieve and the preconditions in which our body is to carry it out, in the case of weight loss, the main objective is to achieve ketosis and thus begin to lose that localized fat without having loss of muscle mass, we must also have knowledge of how to break the fast, and this step must be done gradually, that is to say, to break the fast they must consume slowly the foods, it is advisable to begin with a broth of bones for example, and is that with the practice of the fast also you can determine which are the possible foods that produce inflammation to you, since after having a period of time without consuming foods and to begin gradually to ingest them, you can determine if some of them produces discomfort to you, for example, or inflammation in your organism.

Whether for weight loss or any other purpose, it is necessary to remember that we must break the fast with a balanced diet and within the ketogenic diet because otherwise, everything achieved with fasting would be lost.

When we apply fasting in any of the cases explained above, one of the first things that occur is that the levels of sugar and insulin in the blood decrease, it is observed that it increases the body's response to insulin, which is the hormone that regulates blood sugar levels, therefore regulating these levels begins to burn that localized fat that we all want to eliminate from our body.

Fasting also increases the production of growth hormone, adrenaline, and glucagon, which are responsible for activating the mechanism of lipolysis, which is the combustion of fats, thus helping to eliminate body fat while preserving the muscles. It is a type of food in which there is no hunger, and excellent results are obtained.

After two to three weeks of limiting carbohydrate intake to less than 50 grams per day and applying fasting you start to observe how blood sugar levels fall, it is advisable to also consume salt in meals to prevent some of the side effects. When fasting is done there are periods of keto-adaptation that is generally achieved between two to four weeks, there are studies that classify the keto-adaptation in three phases, the short phase of adaptation that is achieved from 7 to 14 days, the medium phase that is achieved from 14 to 35 days of fasting, and the long phase of adaptation that is achieved from 2 to 12 months. In the process of keto-adaptation, what can be observed is a considerable decrease in symptoms caused by carbohydrate restrictions, when a keto-adaptation process is being carried out, the body feels more energetic, the body is already detoxified, and the changes and benefits in our body are beginning to be noticed.

Fasting has the particularity that can be chosen in an open way, that is, yourselves can choose what type of fast to choose, what type of food you should consume and when you should consume, this makes it a method to lose weight quite flexible, and in fact, by being able to be applied in this way and not be a strict diet has been achieved that more and more people are applying it successfully.

It is a good method to achieve slimming and increase fat burning and is that when the body reaches ketosis, the body is responsible for taking the fat accumulated from our body and thus burns the fat we have accumulated. In the case of training done on a fast, there are opinions that suggest that it is good to exercise on a fast because on a fast the body has fewer amounts of glucose and in this way it uses fat to acquire the energy demanded by exercise, in fact, there are studies that have shown that exercising on a fast burns more fat than doing it after eating. Although exercising on fasting is good, it is also recommended not to do high-intensity exercises. Again it is recommended that these practices are performed in a controlled manner by trained people. Not everyone can apply fasting, not everyone can exercise fasting, it is necessary to carefully evaluate the individual capacities of each person to implement these protocols, what is certain is that great benefits have been observed when applying them and that in the case of weight loss the results have been quite encouraging, moreover, all these methods to lose weight depend mainly on perseverance and planning to perform them, it is necessary and advisable to consume supplements, vitamins, minerals, electrolytes, in conjunction with the implementation of fasting and ketogenic diets.

CHAPTER 9:
FOOD INCLUDED ON INTERMITTENT FASTING

In order to know what types or which foods are included or allowed when fasting, we must know what kind of fasting we will perform. However, the foods do not change a lot according to the fasting of our preference. So, we will give you an example of the food included in the 16/8 fasting

What is Intermittent Fasting 16/8 Based on?

This type of intermittent fasting is very simple and only consists of dividing our day "meal plan" in two, of which 8 hours will be in those we are allowed to eat, and 16 hours will be the hours in which our body will be fasting.

Usually, these 16 hours of fasting include the hours of sleep, so it is easier to do this without being fully aware of the time we spend fasting.

We can present a very simple case describing the lifestyle of a person who carries out this diet, this person in his intermittent diet 16/8 gets up at 8:00 AM to do their physical activity such as cardio for 45 minutes, then makes his first meal at 12:00 pm (from here starts the 8 hours) until 8 pm, when eats his dinner and after two hours goes to sleep. If we count his night hours, we can see that this person is able to take a light fast which is not reflected in such a heavy way.

One of the great advantages of this diet is the ease of adapting it to our lifestyle, so we do not become so complicated a task to be able to maintain a proper diet.

How Can I Organize My Intermittent Fasting Schedules?

How we will make our approach to the 16/8 method of the intermittent diet, we will propose a series of schedules with which we can govern ourselves initially, but these will always depend on our agenda and ability to fulfill them.

We will have as a first option the most used: This 8-hour diet starts from 10:00 in the morning and ends at 6:00 pm, entering a period of fasting from 6:00pm to 10: 00 am, thus having our 16 hours of fasting.

As a second option, we will have the previously explained where the first meal begins at 12:00 pm, having as last meal dinner at 8:00 pm.

As a third option, we have the case in which the first meal is at 1:00 pm, being the last meal at 9:00 pm.

Can Fasting Cause Hunger Attacks?

Many times the fear factor of people when fasting is the fear of "suffering from hunger," which generates anxiety so strong that they could end up eating even worse than they should.

Well, this is a myth, because at the moment each meal arrives we learn to enjoy more and we can even feel satisfied with each bite without having to exceed ourselves.

However, to avoid having such cravings during fasting hours, it is essential that each meal contains nutritious foods so that we can get that feeling of being satisfied. In case we come to present an episode of anxiety or craving the most advisable is to drink a glass of water or alternatively a vegetable broth to soothe a little, there will come the point at which we get used and can even favor us in complementing our food dishes.

Does Coffee Break the State of Fasting?

- Up to now, no data has been found to confirm that drinking coffee can take us out of the fasting state. Even many experts include coffee in the diet or fasting regime (as long as this is coffee alone, without any "topping" or sugar)

However, there are cases of people who prefer to avoid coffee and resort to options such as homemade broths of vegetables, water and salt, sugarless gum, and even drink a lot of water. All this is acceptable as long as we avoid soft drinks (with or without sugar) and packaged juices.

Can I Eat Anything Once my Fasting Hours Are Over?

Once our fasting hours are over, the ideal is to eat (and drink) as healthily as possible, as it is useless to fast if we do not eat properly.

In the case of fasting, it is recommended to follow the Harvard dish model. What is this?

This is just one way to serve our food. It will be as follows: The main part of our plate (which will contain half of it) will be vegetables; a quarter will be carbohydrates, the other quarter will be meats (red or white such as fish, chicken) or legumes.

With this, we seek that the heaviest of our foods are vegetables and carbohydrates, and proteins are the companions of our meals.

Additionally, if we want a dessert, we recommend fruit, fruit salad, or yogurt, always avoiding those quick snacks that are not of natural origin.

What Foods Are Recommended for the Permitted Feeding Hours?

Really there is no diet by which we must regulate ourselves in a mandatory way since it is considered that with fasting, we are burning the necessary calories. However, it is always good to maintain a properly balanced diet so that these lost calories can be noticeable in the long term in our body.

Mostly it is recommended the consumption of fresh foods such as vegetables and fruits. This way, we are starting with a better lifestyle through food. The amounts of protein and even the same fresh food should be provided by a nutritionist as it will help us improve certain aspects based on what our body needs.

How Many Meals Per Day?

Usually, when making this type of diet, you have 2 or 3 main meals, and even in some cases, there are people who make a small snack (as long as it is within the hours in which the intake of food is allowed).

- If a person usually wakes up late, they can start the day with lunch, have a mid-afternoon mini snack and finally close with dinner.

There are other cases of morning people starting their day with a full breakfast, lunch, and dinner/snack.

Next, we are going to see an example of a menu that could serve us as a base to adapt our menu, according to our needs:

Intermediate Fasting 16/8: Morning Option

If you are one of those persons who start their day very early, you will need enough energy to perform in your daily tasks, so this is the option that can best suit you.

In this option, you will be able to eat food only from 10:00 am to 6:pm (18:00h), the rest of the time our body will be in a state of fasting:

- 7:00 am Start the day with tea, coffee, infusion, or water.
- 10:00 am First meal, full breakfast.
- 2:00 pm (14:00 hrs): Lunch
- 6:00pm (18:00 hrs): Snack or dinner
- 8:00 pm (20:00 hrs): In case of anxiety, hunger, or cravings, you can prepare a vegetable broth or some tea.

If you are one of those persons who love to sleep and start their day a little later than usual, you should be very attentive to what are your mealtimes and to be able to meet everything at the time, so this is the option that can best suit you.

In this option you will be able to eat only from 12:00 am to 8:pm (20:00h), the rest of the time our body will be in a state of fasting:

- 9:00 am Start the day with tea, coffee, infusion, or water.
- 12:00 am First meal; this must be a complete lunch to be able to contribute all the necessary energies.
- 3:00 pm (14:00 hrs): snack
- 6:00pm (18:00 hrs): dinner
- 8:00 pm (20:00 hrs): In case of anxiety, hunger, or cravings, you can prepare a vegetable broth or some tea.

HOW LONG IS IT RECOMMENDED TO CONTINUE WITH THE INTERMITTENT FASTING ROUTINE?

The most recommendable thing is to follow this regime until we obtain the changes that we look for to obtain in our organism and body. Nevertheless, we must not forget that also to obtain these results we have to exercise constantly.

Similarly, it is not totally forbidden that we can give ourselves a pleasure (dessert, pizza, hamburger, soda, etc.) from time to time.

We cannot forget an important complement. Do some physical activity:

In order to achieve the desired weight (and even physical endurance) is very important to exercise at least 3 times a week, so the effects of fasting will be more noticeable.

If we want to do physical activity during the 16 hours of fasting, we can only take the following:

- Water
- Tea
- Infusions
- Coffee (no sugar)
- Vegetable broth (preferably shredded)

If you are very anxious, you may be able to calm your anxiety with sugar-free gum.

These drinks are okay as long as they don't contain sugar, sweeteners, vegetables, milk, or anything else that may contain calories.

So, when fasting, there is no forbidden food or a list of food that is allowed, but the food you eat after fasting will mean a lot to get the results you are looking for. In order to get the best results, it is strongly recommended to eat using the keto diet after fasting. We will discuss how these two methods are related in the following chapter.

CHAPTER 10:
INTERMITTENT FASTING AND KETO DIET

The ketogenic diet, as we appreciated in previous chapters, has a great number of benefits for the organism. It is a very popular feeding method nowadays and in which the fundamental purpose for which it is used is to lose weight.

As we already know with the low-carbohydrate diet, without consuming processed sugar and other conditions that carry the keto eating plan, different levels of ketosis can be reached, which finally, for people who do it in an adequate and disciplined way, is what they hope to reach.

Added to this, is intermittent fasting, which is a complement to the keto diet because it has been proven that people who apply it together reach ketosis faster.

Now, some people have managed to confuse this plan with the fact of going hungry, and in fact it is not recommended that this happens, to reach the levels of ketosis it is not necessary to go hungry or consume the already known "keto cravings", the fundamental thing is to avoid carbohydrate-rich foods such as cereals, sugars, legumes, rice, potatoes, sweets, of course, juices and most fruits.

The standard ketogenic diet is a diet plan that is characterized by being very low in carbohydrates, with a moderate intake of protein and high in fat. It normally contains 75% fat, 20% protein, and only 5% carbohydrates. As we already know if all these requirements are met blood sugar levels can be reduced and insulin levels too, and this way there will be a transition in the metabolism of the body in which carbohydrates are replaced as energy source for the body by fats and ketones, thus reaching the main objective which is "ketosis". When the insulin levels fall, ketones are manufactured, and this can be noticed in the second, third or fourth week. This period is known as Keto-adaptation (KA). The body becomes dependent on sugar as the main fuel ((glycogen) to depend mainly on fat and for this to be achieved, we must overcome the keto-adaptation phase.

When we finally change our main fuel we are going to have an unlimited fuel for fat to which people with other types of diet do not have access, and on the other hand, we are going to have glycogen as a secondary fuel, And that is how our body must actually work, because we are able to store 2000kcal of glycogen but more than 1,000,000 kcal of fat safely so we can store energy for ourselves.

For a person who must consume 2000 kcal daily it is achieved with the keto diet in the following way:

70-80%, which are equivalent to 1400-1600 kcal of fat, 15-25%, which corresponds to 300-500 kcal of protein, 5% of carbohydrates, which corresponds to approximately 100 kcal. More or less, we would be talking about 150-170 grams of fat per day, 75-125 grams of protein per day, and 25 grams of carbohydrates per day approximately.

But all these amounts are easy to get if we eat naturally, if we get our meals to be based mainly on meat, fish especially oily fish, egg, cheese, cream, all kinds of vegetables and this opens a large window of food, mushrooms, nuts, seeds, MCT oil, coconut oil, olive oil preferably extra virgin, butter or ghee, fruits such as avocado, coconut, berries, strawberries, blueberries, blackberries,. Basically, eat unprocessed food and processed organic from natural preference, but each of us will be able to structure our eating plan in the way we consider most appropriate.

Within ketosis, we have the term known as "nutritional ketosis", which is nothing more than consuming foods that do not depend on fat or protein, in order to reach the metabolic state called ketosis, we simply must completely and absolutely eliminate sugar, wheat and its derivatives and lower to its minimum expression the simple carbohydrates, and eliminate in its entirety the complex carbohydrates, which are commonly known as processed foods, bread, pasta, hamburger, etc..

In this way what is going to happen is that in your organism the glucose reserves are going to be depleted, and the ketogenic bodies will begin to feed, to look for energies of that accumulated fat in your body that we so much want to eliminate and it is there where you begin to feel the ketogenic state or ketosis. In fact, a high fat-burner in a natural way is the intermittent fasting practiced in a responsible and supervised way. If it is applied correctly, the consumption of artificial burners that we find in the different national and international markets is not necessary, so it is only a matter of organization and discipline, and you will begin to experience all the changes in your body and in your health. An exact way to determine if you are already in Ketosis is with a simple blood test, currently in the same way that there are devices on the market that have the ability to measure blood sugar levels, there are also several brands that can measure the levels of ketones in your body, so you can acquire any of them and thus keep track and know when you have reached the optimal level of ketosis.

However, when you stop consuming sugar and carbohydrates, you will mainly start a detoxification process, as the body begins to eliminate all that amount of anti-nutrients that for so long have been allowed into your body and has also damaged your cellular environment. When this detoxification process begins, you will suffer a series of unfriendly symptoms known as " abstinence syndrome," in this case, you will begin to experience the following symptoms:

- Sleeping difficulties.
- Apathy and listlessness.
- Symptoms of depression.
- Irritable attitude.
- Appetite disturbances.
- Lethargy.
- Anxiety.
- Thirst.

All these symptoms mentioned are due to your body starts to suffer the " abstinence syndrome " because you have restricted your body of carbohydrates and sugars, but before the appearance of these symptoms we have some recommendations that you can do when you feel that way:

- Drink plenty of water,
- It is recommended to drink apple vinegar, prepared as follows, dilute one tablespoon of vinegar in 4 ounces of water each morning on an empty stomach.

- And the most important recommendation is to eat well, it is not necessary as previously recommended to go hungry. Since once this stage is over, everything will be easier.

The important thing is to eat within the allowed requirements, but without going hungry, in fact you will notice that once your body has finally been detoxified and cleaned, your body begins to change and you begin to learn to listen to your body, and this means that when you eat a food that is harmful or alters your cellular environment, it will indicate with discomfort that you should not eat that food. In addition, you will have better absorption of nutrients because your digestive system improves, being one of the most important benefits of this diet since the intestine is currently considered as the second brain.

Now, as for fasting, we already know all the benefits involved in applying it, and the most important is that it is a potential fat burner for our body, helps reduce cellulite, among other great benefits that we already know. But fasting means not to eat and the intermittent fasting means not to eat for a period of time. It could be daily, weekly or monthly as you wish to apply it.

What will break your fast? Food. Fasting will promote the autophagy or recycling process of damaged cellular components, and large benefits of fasting are directly related to autophagy. But this process occurs gradually and will depend on our particular organism. It will depend on each tissue whether neurons, liver, muscle, immune system, intestines, and yes, the whole body in general.

There are studies that relate exercise, diet, and fasting with autophagy. All this process takes time; the changes are not going to happen overnight. First, the body must go through a process of adaptation.

In autophagy, the cell needs energy, and with the implementation of fasting and in the absence of exogenous food, the destruction of damaged internal contents begins, and autophagy begins. In this case, the cells will devour or consume parts of themselves to eliminate viruses, bacteria and all the damage caused by cellular aging and at the same time, obtain fuel to improve their processes.

This process is fundamental for the organism because if it is not carried out, it will lead to inflammatory processes, infectious diseases, Alzheimer's, Parkinson's and cancer. The autophagy achieved or stimulated through fasting is an intelligent way for the body to detoxify itself in a natural way since the cells themselves know what they need and what they don't need for their growth and evolution. Intermittent fasting eliminates toxins, stimulates the immune system, regulates inflammation and promotes longevity.

Generally, the intermittent fast that is performed is 16-8, this method 16/8 is known as "Leangains" method, with this modality you will consume food for 8 hours, and you will fast for 16 hours. If you wish, you can include within the 16 hours of fasting the period of sleep, so that it is easier and bearable this period of intermittent fasting. If you apply it in this way the most common is to lengthen breakfast at noon or what would be lunch, and finally your second meal of the day corresponds to the dinner, at night before 8 pm. This is an easy way to apply intermittent fasting daily accompanied by the keto diet, and if you can also if you can add exercise, you will love the final results.

And it is that the intermittent fast is more than a simple restriction of calories, it also produces alterations in the hormones of our body so that they can make better use of their fat reserves. By lowering insulin levels produces a better burning of fat. The secretion of growth hormone increases and, therefore, accelerates the synthesis of protein and using the fat that is available as a source of energy. So that is not only burning fat, but it is also building muscle mass more quickly as if you consume as athletes do. What a wonderful piece of news, isn't it? all that your body is capable of doing naturally if you just take the time to eat properly.

Now, how we should break with that fast?, or how we will have break-fast?, and is that one of the classic ways to break the fast is with the famous "bone broth", preferably homemade, but an hour before breaking the fast is recommended to drink a glass of soda water; it can be with cinnamon or apple vinegar, salt or lemon, this drink will help you prepare your stomach digestive enzymes that have been without food for 16 hours with only water and coffee, if you consume this drink it is likely that the food can be absorbed without stomach problems and absorbing all the nutrients to the maximum. After this, we can consume the bone broth, which is a liquid food will not force our stomach to work with heavy food, but rather easy digestion apart from the bone broth is rich in fat, protein, and vitamins. And an hour later you can eat a plate of solid food under the requirements of the keto diet, which you already know widely, this is a way to break the fast in a way suitable for your body, and to quickly reach ketosis and autophagy.

CHAPTER 11:
SPECIFIC BENEFITS FOR YOUR HEALTH

When we observe the normal functioning of human beings, we can see that the body feeds on glucose, which is the molecule that is generated by the consumption of carbohydrates and sugars, but an excessive consumption of them, could cause damage to our health, such as becoming diabetics, which is a disease that occurs when glucose is produced in excess, and the body is not able to use it, having an excess of glucose in the blood, so to speak, causing problems in our organs, also, an excess consumption of carbohydrates can generate overweight, leading us, in the long run to very serious diseases, such as could be, the diabetes mentioned above.

Therefore, it could be said that this way of eating is not the best for our body, since the consumption of carbohydrates, either in a normal amount, the organs of our body do not always interact well with glucose, because having high levels of it in our body, insulin levels are also increased, and it has direct implications on the functioning of our body, so that it could even alter our metabolism.

Due to these reasons, we managed to achieve the state of ketosis, which is a state of our body, in which in a normal state, is a large consumption of fat, segregating a molecule called ketone, being this the main source of food for our body, or better said, is a source of energy extremely efficient and good for our body, which can produce side effects, not necessarily bad.

This function is essential for personal survival, since because of this, people can have an alternate source of energy, since at the time we run out of glucose, the body will proceed to consume their energy reserves produced by the ketone, of course, this energy reserve is not infinite, because the same may last a few days, therefore, this process is very important to continue with brain function in an effective way, because the process of storing glucose is very ineffective in our body, for that reason, we prefer to do the ketogenic feeding, because our body evolved to survive for several days, perhaps even weeks, being this an extremely extreme case, because the person is already trained to do this, not anyone is able to do such a task. Therefore, we could say that the process of ketosis is responsible for ensuring that the brain is feeding properly, in the event that you do not have enough glucose to feed it, and does so, as we explained previously, through the deposits of fat.

We can see that ketones interact in a better way with our organs, especially with our brain, since with this combination, the processes of the same can be carried out in a more optimal way. And as we should know, or at least intuit it, the brain is the organ that consumes more energy, therefore, to have a good ketone-brain relationship, we can say that our body is able to work better than with glucose, and is not that our brain works with fat, no, but with the molecules that segregate the liver, product of high fat consumption and low carbohydrate consumption, therefore, the brain proceeds to work with the ketones, thus achieving a more efficient consumption of energy, moreover, we assume that you have suffered episodes in your life in which you feel exhausted, without the need to have done many exercises or many activities, a possible reason for this condition, is that your body is poorly alimented, because your body is not generating much glucose or is not processing it well, by this we mean, to having a high level of glucose in the blood, insulin levels rise, and people feel a certain tiredness, a palpable example is that when you eat a large plate of pasta, immediately after you feel tired and sleepy, this is due to the fact that your insulin levels are high, producing a state of heaviness in your body, but in the case that you do or practice another type of diet, you will feel more energy, furthermore, there are people who, with only the ketogenic diet, have managed to fast for long periods of time, without feeling short of energy, thus having a better performance of our body, concluding that our brain, when it sees the opportunity to feed on ketones produced by the consumption of fat, feels more energy, indeed, there are people who certify that when they changed their habits, they started to feel more energetic, and if this was not enough, they also felt better mentally focused, so we cannot say that this diet is not only responsible for losing weight but physically benefit our body.

But, we are going to go step by step, therefore we will explain little by little the benefits of the consumption of a good ketogenic diet for our body, which can even improve the state of the heart of our body, due to this reason, we invite you to migrate from food diet, of course, if you wish, since you will be able to observe in a fast way the improvement in your health.

As we already know, the ketogenic diet has many benefits for people who consume it, they can go from improving the brain condition of patients, to improve respiratory problems of people, for that reason, they are not only needed to lose weight but also for some pathologies that you may have and want to solve.

The first benefit that it provides us, is as well it is known, the decrease of the weight, this result is obtained thanks to that the keto diet, is in charge of burning the fat and in this process of burning it is entered into ketosis, coming this way to lose a great number of kilograms, obtaining a better health in the people who suffer from obesity. When achieving the goal of coming out of the obesity state, the following benefits can be obtained:

- Reduces the possibility of death, as obesity is the leading cause of death in the United States.
- The possibility of suffering from diseases such as cancer, diabetes, heart attacks, gallstones.
- Many people who are overweight feel a lot of depression because of the shape of their body, and when they get out of it, these people improve their mental health, thus increasing their quality of life.
- There are many people who, because they are overweight, do not sleep very well for different reasons, but the main reason is sleep apnea, which is a cause closely related to overweight, which can cause high blood pressure or even heart attacks.

As we can already see, reducing our body weight can significantly improve our quality of life since overweight affects us in many areas of health, and not only the visual that is also important, but it can affect us so much that it can lead to death.

We can also find a direct relationship between the ketogenic diet and the health of the heart, because as we explained previously, this type of food, allows a rapid loss of body fat index, therefore, allow us to quickly lose weight, because it burns fat in an exaggerated form so to speak, thus achieving a more than considerable reduction in cardiovascular risks, because they have a close relationship with obesity, because if the person is obese, then it has more chances of having heart disease, coupled with this, being obese implies that you have a high blood pressure, which could cause a heart attack, which can be fulminant or not. On the other hand reduces the amount of cholesterol in our body, which indicates that we have a large amount of fat in our blood, and having such a condition can also cause some of our arteries to block, which can also lead to a heart attack. For these reasons, we recommend doing the low-carbohydrate diet, so as to achieve reduce these pathologies and clean our body of fats found in our blood, thus achieving a better protection of our blood system thereby preventing this type of disease, otherwise, also when practicing the ketogenic diet, we achieve a cell cleaning in our blood, throwing harmful toxins into our body, due to the process of increased autophagy, which, as we said previously cleanses our body, and there is nothing better than having the body clean, because having our body so, we can begin to see it work better or improve its functioning by cleaning ourselves internally, since our body will work as new, without any impediment. But said all this, and explained that this diet reduces cholesterol and all of the above, you may wonder: why make a high-fat diet low cholesterol if I was banned from fried chicken, and this is no more than fried protein? Well, it is not that all fats are good, on the contrary, there is nothing more harmful than some fried foods, for that reason it is not a very good practice to eat them, but what is true, is that you can consume many fats, as long as they are good fats from nature, such as avocado fat, or natural peanut butter.

As if that were not enough, the keto diet, not only helps the heart, but to an accumulation of other organs, another very important one, I would not know if I could tell you that the most important in the body, but if the one that consumes the most energy, such as the brain, the first thing we can say about the relationship of the ketogenic diet with the brain, is that in one of the first cases that the keto diet was implemented, it was in a patient suffering from epilepsy, which indicates that the patient suffered from constant convulsions, and by prescribing a diet low in carbohydrates, but higher in fat, a considerable improvement could be observed. Then, we can say that studies have been done on people who suffer from epilepsy, and the results conclude that this diet does help them, but it, is recommended more frequently to children, since it is easier to guide a child who is going to eat or not, and also the brain of the adult is already fully formed. The results are very positive, since at least half of the children to whom the test was applied, stopped suffering epileptic seizures, and another amount, even more than fifty percent, since here we also count those who did not suffer their epileptic seizures anymore, but those who had their frequency of epileptic seizures considerably reduced, therefore, we cannot be one hundred percent conclusive, saying that it ends with epilepsy or something like that, but there is something that we can say, and it is that the results are hopeful for a bright future, in the field of epilepsy. Also, the same diet can be used for those who suffer from Alzheimer's, since it is a degenerative disease, which causes people to gradually lose their memory, until the time comes when they can remember almost nothing, becoming so complicated the situation that can lead to the death of patients with the disease. We can say that the results are positive, it is because first, the experiments carried out on animals, were positive, since the mice which had certain brain degeneration, were given ketogenic food, and it was possible to obtain, first, that they managed to regenerate parts of their brains, and second, because it has also been achieved that the ketogenic food manages to improve the connections between the axons and dendrite, thus obtaining better communication between neurons, obtaining a brain more capable of performing any kind of tasks.

So, what we can say with this, is that we recommend you feed yourself with ketogenic food, because as you could have seen, not only helps us to reduce our weight, but we can improve a large accumulation of health conditions, improving the lives of our heart, improving our respiratory system or even reactivating some brain connections.

It is important to highlight the fact that the food used in the keto diet, such as fish and other seafood, has a lot of omega 3 and other components that are scientifically proven to have positive effects on brain functioning, performance, and memory.

CHAPTER 12:
SLEEP, STRESS, AND MINDSET

Have you ever felt so stressed that you couldn't sleep? Many times those sleeping difficulties or insomnia are caused naturally in response to the levels of stress we may be under; in fact, sometimes, when we have trouble falling asleep, they can cause stress.

It is known that our mind has immense power when it is not calm, it directly affects the body, and it may be difficult for us to calm both in this type of situation.

Since we are young, we have used the word to say that we are stressed, but what is stress really?

We can define stress as the set of physiological reactions that are presented to us when we are suffering a state of nervous tension caused by various situations, whether anxiety, overwork, traumatic situations to which we have been exposed.

In this way, stress is directly associated with emotional distress and body tension. These when they increase their levels of excitement, which alert the body to prepare to face the possible danger to which we submit.

DIFFERENT TYPES OF STRESS

- Common Stress: They are the natural reactions that occur in our organism to certain situations, which we can define as stressful. Many times these types of stress are anxieties about something we are going to be under, and this natural reaction can help us overcome such situations.
- Workplace stress: This happens when the demands on our work environment are so huge that they cause us to collapse into harmful emotional and physical reactions to which our ability to solve a problem is not possible to solve.
- Pathological stress: This occurs when the stress we have is presented in an intense way for a prolonged period, which could cause us psychological and

physical problems, causing anxiety crisis, crying crisis, depression, and many other physical alterations that turn this into chronic and constant stress.

- Post-traumatic stress: This is the stress that occurs after a person has lived through an event that significantly affected them, whether it was a traffic accident or a natural disaster. As a consequence of this trauma, the person often has thoughts that cause terror. This type of stress occurs at any age but is mostly the result of childhood experiences.

Many times, the way in which we see ourselves in the world can influence these reactions of the body (just as the mind can betray us and make the situation look much worse, generating more anxiety).

This is why if we feel stressed or not, has a direct relationship with how we perceive things, for example, imagine that we have a very common case of everyday life which could be leading us to very high levels of stress:

In this case, we have to pay a household utility bill for $100, and we have two cases:

1. A person who has $1,000 in his account and pays that bill does not affect his budget.
2. A person who has $60 in his account and pays that bill would cost him a little bit because he would have to collect a little more and put aside any extra problems that affect his budget.

In these cases, we could observe how one person would find this situation totally normal, while another person could generate very great anguish and perceives more significantly the problem that is presented because his ability to evaluate the resources and face the problem could have a great impact on their mood.

If we look at stress as a way of trying to balance the demands of life and the resources we have to deal with it, we have two options:

1. Reduce the demands we perceive
2. Seek ways to increase our available resources.

It is important to emphasize that not always resources are limited to a monetary value, our resources could also make references to cognitive things such as improving our behavior, lifestyle, a way of thinking, skills to control our emotions, take control of some situation, have faith and even physical aspects such as improving our endurance and energy.

If we feel that we are facing a stress episode, we must ask ourselves the following questions in order to find a possible immediate solution; what is the factor that generates stress? What are the resources I have to solve this problem? How can I apply these resources to the solution of my problem?

Many times we focus more on the problem without taking into account that we have the solution in our hands. That is why before altering ourselves, we must think coldly about why the situation is happening, and in this way, we will be avoiding a worse result.

STRESS IN OUR BODY

Our body reacts to stress when the hormones that cause it are released; these cause our body to be attentive to any problem that might occur, this causes our body muscles to tension and thus progressively increase our heart rate.

This type of reaction could be interpreted as the way in which our body protects itself from any approaching danger and can even help us make quick decisions in any situation. The problem occurs when chronic stress occurs because our body will remain alert to any event even if we are not close to danger, and in the long term, could significantly affect our health.Chronic stress may cause us:

- Acne
- Menstrual problems
- High Blood Pressure
- Cardiac insufficiency
- Depression or anxiety
- Obesity

In addition to directly affecting health, it can influence our daily activities, or physical problems that we don't realize are caused by stress. These can be:

- Headaches.
- Lack of energy or concentration.
- Diarrhea.
- Constipation.
- Poor memory.
- Trouble sleeping.
- Sexual problems.
- Discomfort in the stomach.
- Need to use alcohol to feel temporarily distracted.
- Weight loss or gain

Sleeping is one of the resources which help to decrease stress in a considerable way, it helps us to cognitive processes such as good memory, concentration, and attention, it helps to the good psychological and emotional functioning since many times when a person does not rest enough he is in a bad mood and in this way he expresses his bad attitude towards the world.

Sleeping properly helps us recharge physical energy, improve injuries, and even growth.

Sleep is influenced by the body clock system and the dream controller. These are responsible for determining when to rest and for how long we should do it or for how long our body needs it.

If we have the correct functioning of our system, the one in charge of promoting the state of sleep will have power over our alert system every night. Unlike if we get to have a very high level of stress when resting, our system that is responsible for promoting the alerts of our body will have greater power over the system that promotes sleep, causing insomnia or difficulties to fall asleep.

Ideal advice to reduce the levels of stress that we may present when we go to bed to sleep:

If you feel too anxious to be able to promote sleep, you can get out of bed, drink a glass of water and try to relax your mind.

Plan a relaxing hour before going to bed: It is important that before going to bed, we have an hour to devote ourselves to bathing, relaxation stretching, and even reading. These simple exercises can relax our body from any problem that we have presented in the day.

The bed is a place to rest: It is important to avoid any type of activity that generates stress (tasks, work, fighting).

ADVICE TO BE ABLE TO LOOK FOR EASY SOLUTIONS TO OUR WORRIES

- Develop routines and habits: Performing physical activities and even eating a healthy diet can help our mind to clear and even improve our body clock.
- Self-care: It is important to spend time doing any type of activity that helps us mentally and makes us feel good. Many times we try to solve a problem without feeling good, and this is very important because it affects us emotionally and we will not have the energy to deal with another problem.
- Knowing our personal strengths: It is important to know the way we see ourselves. In this way, our problem-solving abilities could increase significantly when we know what we are capable of facing.
- Relaxation: It is important from time to time to take relaxation breaths to purify our body and connect it with the mind. A clean mind can think more clearly to an overwhelmed mind.
- Connect with others: It is important to receive support, and we achieve this by surrounding ourselves with our loved ones, so we know that we are not alone against the world. Many studies indicate that surrounding ourselves with loved ones can have a great influence on our physical and psychological health.

TIPS TO LESSEN OUR WORRIES:

Organization: It is important to dedicate at least one hour a day to be able to take care of everything that could worry us or could become a worry in the future. In this way, we will be able to obtain a better level of relaxation at night. It is advisable to write down everything. In this way, we do not overlook anything, and so we slowly go thinking about how to solve them (either present problem, something that has not happened or that we imagine a possible scenario which will not exist).

Thought: Our mind is a powerful weapon and from it can depend on our state of mind and even what we are capable of doing, to be able to do this we just have to put aside the negative thoughts and concentrate on the positive ones.

Many times we get involved in a negative scenario believing that we will never get out of that gap, but the reality is that you can, and everything depends on us, let's put the concerns aside and deal with it without fear of failing or at least trying.

Organizing our time: This is a very effective way to prevent future stress. Organizing our priorities is the most important thing because we avoid overlooking something and being always in order we can perform our daily tasks much faster.

Communication: Communicating our concerns or asking for some help is never too much. We do not know if we have a problem, and another subject has the solution (as the very known phrase states: Two heads think better than one). When we reduce the number of demands we have, our stress levels decrease dramatically.

Identify and communicate how we feel: Another effective way to prevent future stress may be to identify how we are feeling at that moment, whether we are going through a difficult time, or have had a discussion that may upset us. In these cases, it is advisable to go to a specialist, a friend or write our feelings on a piece of paper.

At This Point, We Must be Asking Ourselves: How Does This and the Keto Diet Relates? As we have seen before, it is well known that in order to follow a diet, we must adapt ourselves and our body to certain habits to which we may not have been used to. This will always be the key when it comes to any kind of diet because if we do not have the right mentality, we will not succeed in trying to adapt our body to it.

As human beings, we will always follow a pattern that has never failed since we were very small. Whenever we discover something new (in this case the keto diet), we get excited and set out to meet every goal needed to achieve the goal we have set for ourselves; over time we will notice the changes we have obtained as a result of the effort to accomplish certain rules. The problem comes when we have reached this objective, and we stop obeying strictly the rules (which led us to this objective).

In the case of the keto diet, we will need to strictly comply with all the steps, since in this way our body will begin to make certain changes and will need a period of adaptation to be able to receive these changes in a good way.

Many times, people who try to do this diet fail to see the promising results that everyone talks about doing the keto diet and enter a state of despair and stress. Why does this happen, this is for the simple reason that these people do not start with the right mentality, this could apply to any type of diet or feeding regime.

Through the following steps, we will achieve a good motivation and guidance to maintain the right mentality at the time of making this diet (or any other):

STEP 1: START WITH WHAT YOU HAVE

Many times when you start a diet, you feel motivated and start buying food based on a dietary plan that your body has not adapted to.

In most cases, when a person starts a diet or a strict diet is in order to lose weight, which is why it is considered very important to take it easy as you can not change habits drastically without consequences.

The process of our body to adapt to new habits should be gradual, if we start with what we have, we will gradually decrease the foods that do not suit us (as indicated by our specialist in nutrition), and thus our body will be able to assimilate these changes and release the old habits.

If we allow our body to assimilate these changes, we can see how the results are taking place by themselves, such as weight loss and improvement of some aspects of our health and even physical aspects. Unlike if we force our body to a drastic change, which can bring negative consequences such as weight gain or hormonal imbalance.

It is important to remember that the limits can only be set by ourselves, and it depends on how things work. Changes are always good as long as we accept them in a healthy way to ensure the basis for the success of our diet.

So if I do this correctly and start with what I have at home to change my diet, am I going to be successful with this diet?

As we mentioned earlier, before starting a diet, you must go to a nutritionist, and from here, we are going to enter into a kind of experiment in which we can evaluate whether this new style of feeding suits us or not.

Why an experiment? We can say that we submit ourselves to an experiment because we will not know if it will be successful and the diet will adapt to us effectively or cause negative effects, this is a risk to which we must be prepared, and we will begin with what we have to gain confidence as we get to know ourselves better.

It won't matter what level of physical condition we have or our daily routine of eating habits, as long as we feel willing to do something, it will come naturally; don't try hard to buy foods that may not be to your liking. Know yourself, and in this way, the other steps will be easy.

STEP 2: ENJOY YOUR FOOD

This step is directly related to step 1 because when we start with what we have in our kitchen, in a certain way are the foods we like and enjoy, if we eat healthily and at the same time feel comfortable with it. A diet will stop calling diet to become a habit.

Many times we fail because we have the mental chip that a diet is based on foods that we will not enjoy and will let us starve, this is false, we can not force ourselves to eat food that we do not tolerate, although it is clear that not everything will always be to our liking, we must take a good balance and not lean to just the extremes.

We should not be alarmed by this of new foods because it may be that as our system adapts to our new habit, our tastes will also change. At first, it may be very frustrating to put aside many of the foods to which we were used to, but instead of tying ourselves to a non-existent torment, we can go balancing the foods we like and those we don't to make our palate get used to.

It is important that we do not see the change of food as a punishment since, in this way, it can be much more complicated to adapt to a new diet. A change must be something exciting, something that intrigues us; we should not be predisposed to the unknown since the keto diet has many food alternatives that may be in accordance with us.

How can I make the process of adapting to new healthy foods easier if I like to eat unbalanced?

First, we must choose which style of keto diet we are going to follow according to our habits and willingness to respect them, followed by this we adapt the foods according to our tastes.

WHAT HAPPENS IF I DO NOT LIKE ANY FOOD INCLUDED IN THE DIET AND I CANNOT EAT IT?

Nothing at all will happen. We can easily look for an alternative food to replace the one we do not like. With this, we are not looking to change our taste buds, but we are looking for a healthier lifestyle. We must allow ourselves to enjoy the process and the changes, so we can embrace the results (weight loss, hormone regulation, etc.) in a more positive way.

I really like sweets and junk food, can it be the right diet for me?

Here arises the big problem that can suffer 50% of people who want to start the keto diet and do not dare, we know that we will accept a new challenge to which we must make certain sacrifices, among them is that, put aside the sweets and reduce them. This could be considered the only major sacrifice we can make when we start in keto.

It may cost us a little more to adapt to these kinds of changes, as it is not something that is achieved overnight. But we can make sure that by changing our mentality, we can succeed in everything we set out to do (even in the keto diet).

STEP 3: WE CAN DO IT

As mentioned above, it is very normal for us to be motivated when discovering or starting a new diet, and we want to get to the results that other people have gotten through this routine.

Many times these testimonials come with a marketing image to attract more people or consumers, so we will see photos that we could think and say are "perfect" and that we want to get to that point, the goal is not to give up.

Many times people are discouraged and feel they are failing because they have idealized that they will get the same results as other people who have told their experience with the diet, not all bodies react in the same way, there are people who may take a little longer and there are people to whom the results will be noticed instantly, but the key is persistence.

Once we have focused on how the diet should work our way, we can see another picture. Many times the road to the goal can be complicated, but the important thing is to keep insisting (in a healthy way), the best thing we could do is to tell our own version of how we take the diet to stay with the doubt of. How would the keto diet have worked for me?

This step is directly related to trust since we must be able to understand that we are capable of accomplishing anything as long as we are insistent and follow the rules properly. If we start a new project with the mentality that we may not be able to achieve it, we are complicating the road to success.

This is why we must mentally prepare ourselves to achieve success with keto, it may sound like an easy task, but in many cases, it can be complicated because, as we mentioned before, we are looking for "quick results" only for it, there is a long way to achieve it.

Once we have gone through those three steps, we should be or getting used to the keto diet. As we mentioned a lot of times in the previous chapter, this diet has a lot of benefits regarding the brain, health, and organs of the body. This new habit will help us to feel a bit less stressed because our body will perform better. We will have more confidence in ourselves. Hence we will be able to face the troubles easily. As the stress is reduced, and our body is on a perfect balance, sleeping will also improve, since no illness or pain or weakness will interrupt our sleep.

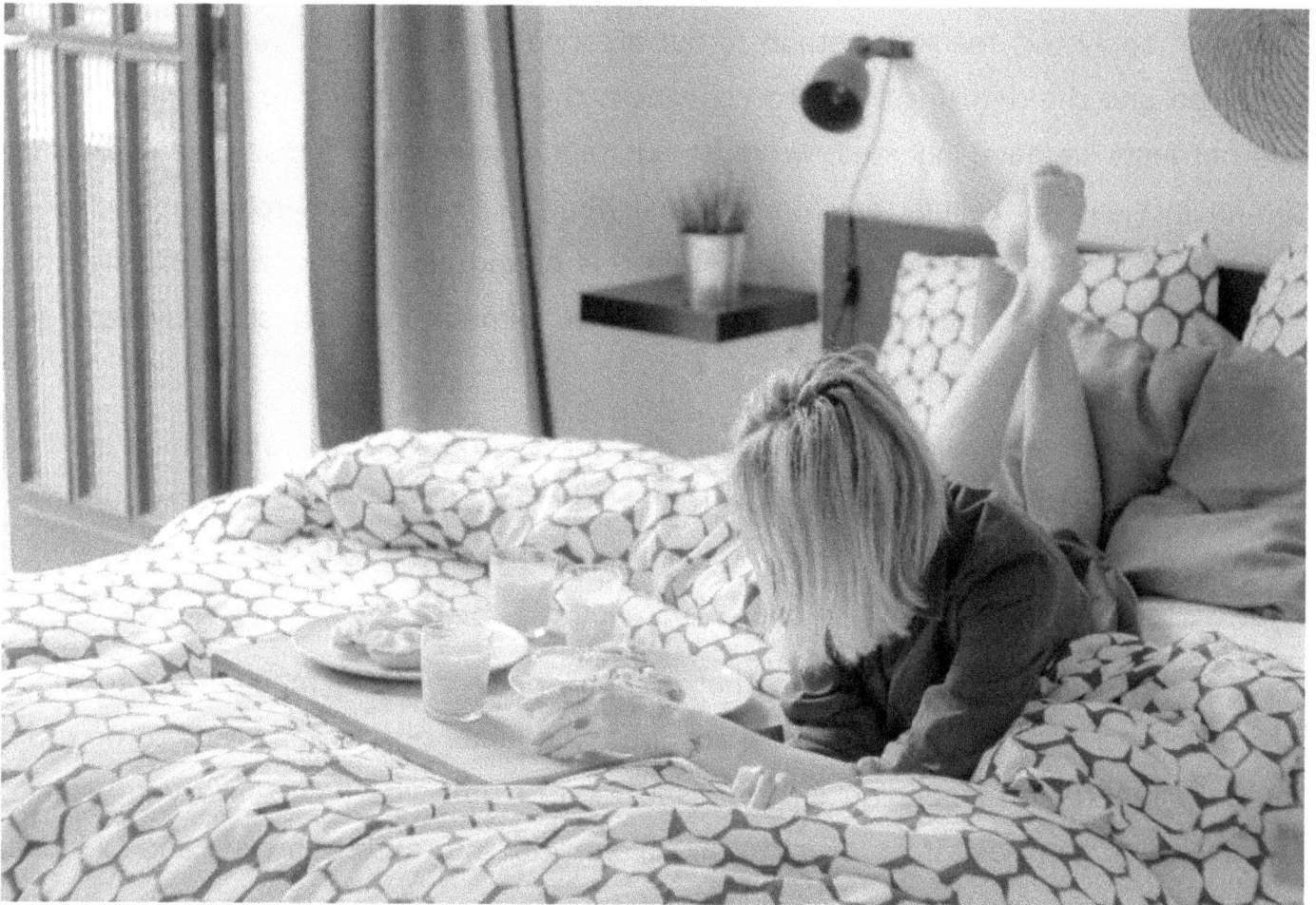

CHAPTER 13:
LIFESTYLE AND DAILY ROUTINE

When we talk about the ketogenic diet, we want more than a diet to be implemented as a discipline and as a lifestyle, since in the case of the ketogenic diet, the long-term changes are those that have an important impact on our health.

When we apply this feeding method to our lifestyle while we start with the metabolic transition and the detoxification process where the body will seek to eliminate all the anti-nutrients we have ingested, we must constantly maintain this discipline so that we can finally clean our cellular environment and when this cellular environment is cleaned and healed it is very important to maintain this eating plan because the moment we return to consume anti-nutrients we return to damage our digestive system and therefore our cellular environment.

That is why it is advisable not to see it in a circumstantial way but rather as a lifestyle where we are learning little by little how to feed ourselves. We will get to know our body, and we will realize that our own body will indicate to us which foods do us harm or which ones we tolerate more and which ones we do not.

If we plan this lifestyle with a routine that we apply daily, it can be made easier to apply, we can plan our menus, and once we acquire experience it is easier for us to program the daily food plan, depending on the disposition of time you have, how you want to make the ketogenic diet if you want to take along with intermittent fasting and exercise, as in fact is commonly recommended to reach faster levels of ketosis and maintain these high levels of energy in our body.

Although many people now think that fat is harmful to health, it happens that with this lifestyle and fat intake we can turn off the fat-storage hormone and thus reprogram our genes to lose weight and burn fat, you are going to notice how the cravings and the desire to eat are reduced because you feel constantly satiated, so not only are you going to lose the kilograms you want, but also, as we have mentioned several times, to improve your health and it is that this should be your main objective and the one that pushes you to take this keto diet as a lifestyle.

The most important ingredient in any meal plan, as the word says is planning, because if we plan, we are not going to be tempted to make bad decisions that may be unhealthy in the end. This is why one of the recommendations we want to make is that at weekends you should take some time to do your weekly planning, your weekly menu, which you can probably alter during the week but to have a more orderly plan you can evaluate what you are going to consume based on the goal you want to achieve.

Start by organizing the dinners, which always turns out to be the most difficult thing to plan, manage, for example, two or three types of vegetables, with a source of proteins complemented of healthy fats always. If you can, add a rich and nutritious salad of vegetables, that way you are arming options of the menu for your week, in the case that your daily life allows it.

The same thing happens with breakfast, you can organize it in a planned way, you can even repeat them without any problem in several opportunities or add other contours to them, assuming that breakfasts are made, because in most cases the ketogenic diet is combined with the known intermittent fast and if it is there, breakfast is suppressed in most cases.

As you can notice everything is a matter of order and planning to make this meal plan a lifestyle, because only then you can get results for longer, and you will notice that as the days go by when you feel energetic, encouraged and in very good health you will not want to leave this lifestyle and your body will thank you.

CHAPTER 14:
KETO RECIPES FOR A GOOD FASTING

We already know the benefits that intermittent fasting brings to our health. We know that it helps to deal with stress and fatigue, delays the signs of aging, helps in the process of hormonal regulation, prevents diseases, improves fat metabolism, controls appetite, and achieves a longer time of autophagy or what is also known as cellular self-regulation.

Fasting helps to control appetite, so when we apply intermittent fasting, it is very easy to carry out a ketogenic diet.

The most important thing about intermittent fasting is that we must eat to break it and the first thing is to consider that as we have so many hours without eating food is not recommended that our first meal is very heavy, but rather it is recommended to break the fast with a liquid diet, and nothing is better than doing it with a broth of bones.

BONE BROTH

Ingredients:

- 1 kg of red beef bones fed on grass.
- Coriander, onion.
- 6 cloves of garlic.
- Salt to taste (preferably Himalayan salt.)
- Apple vinegar.
- Water

Steps to follow:

1.   In a large pot place the bones and enough water leaving about 4 to 5 centimeters to the top of the pot and add the coriander to taste and half chopped onion, only to taste the boiling. Also, add 2 tablespoons of vinegar.

2. Let it rest without lighting the fire for about 20 to 30 minutes as the acid in the vinegar helps the nutrients in the bones become more available.

3. Add enough salt to taste and let cook for about two hours covered, over low heat, and we are alert not to dry our broth

4. It is important to check the broth and remove the foam that is formed above.

5. In the remaining 30 minutes, add more coriander and stir.

MEDALLIONS OF BEEF TENDERLOIN WITH COCONUT

The fusion of the coconut with the meat is an excellent mixture. This is a highly recommended recipe. Coconut, in turn, is an important ally in the ketogenic diet and in intermittent fasting.

Ingredients:

- 1 kg of beef tenderloin, preferably from grass-fed animals.
- 3 spoonfuls of coconut oil.
- 2 cloves of garlic.
- 1 sweet pepper
- 1 large onion.
- 500 ml coconut milk.
- 2 spoonfuls of ground thyme.
- Chicken consommé.
- Pepper to taste.
- Sea salt.

Steps to follow:

1. Let's start seasoning the beef tenderloin with the consommé, a little salt, and pepper, add to taste, and then let it rest for a period of two hours in the refrigerator.

2. Then in a large pot over medium heat, add the coconut oil, and the whole garlic is fried, and when the garlic is browned, we take them out, so we season the oil.

3. Now add the beef tenderloin and seal on both sides. This process can take about 5 minutes.

4. Then we will finely chop the onion along with the paprika and add the thyme and stir several times for flavors to stick.

5. Add the coconut milk, salt, and cover. Let it boil for 30 to 40 minutes or until the loin feels cooked and soft.

6. The sauce will thicken and take a golden tone; this dish should be served hot.

This dish can be served with cauliflower rice or with salads.

CAULIFLOWER CAKE

Ingredients:

- 2 cups cauliflower
- 400 grams of ground beef.
- 4-5 slices of Mozzarella cheese.
- ½ onion
- Sea salt to taste.
- ½ cup whipping cream.

Steps to follow:

1. First, we wash the cauliflower very well. We will add in a pot enough water to boil add the cauliflower for a few minutes until it cooks, it is not recommended to cook for long vegetables, the idea is to cook it al dente. After it is ready, we submerge it in ice water for a few minutes to cut the cooking. Then we strained and reserved.

2. In a frying pan, we are going to fry the onion and the ground meat; we add salt to the taste, pepper if we like.

3. In the blender, pour the whipping cream, salt and add the cauliflower little by little.

4. This way, you will get a kind of mashed potatoes when you finish blending all the cauliflower.

5.   In a lasagne mold, we are going to distribute the ground meat that we prepared previously. We are going to spread it uniformly by all the tray.

6.   On top of this layer, we are going to add the cream that we made with the cauliflower and, finally, a layer with the slices of Mozzarella cheese. We are going to place everything in a uniform way.

7.   Finally, we take it to the oven for 15 minutes until the cheese melts.

When we practice intermittent fasting, one of the advantages we acquire with time and discipline is that we have no appetite because our body acquires a lot of energy. And we are going to feel that. That's why the food that complements fasting is simple but enough for you to feel satisfied. The advisable thing is always to choose natural products, and of good quality, in addition to evaluating the nutritional contributions, the vegetable has that you are going to consume for example. At first, it is probably a bit tedious, but as you acquire experience and knowledge, it becomes easier to organize food plans because one of the objectives we want to achieve is to improve the health of our body.

CHAPTER 15:
RECIPES FOR BREAKFAST AND SNACKS

In a world as dynamic, and as fast as the actual, we can not go around without breakfast, or being hungry over there, unless we are doing some fasting or something like that, as being in a diet already prepared, but in the event that you are not fasting, you cannot walk on your day without breakfast, much less with hunger, for that reason, we recommend, as long as you can, to have breakfast, since this is one of the most important meals of the day, and why not? Sometimes eat a snack at mid-morning or in the afternoon.

BREAKFAST

In this book, we will share two recipes to have a good breakfast, which can feed you adequately, the other breakfasts that you want to eat, you are going to create them, since one of the benefits of the ketogenic diet, is that the recipes are extremely simple.

KETO OMELET

This is a recipe extremely simple and quick to make, many of the people who have prepared such a recipe, say it is better than the classic omelet served in restaurants, because it is spongy and very rich, it allows us to have a variety of ingredients in our omelet, without the need to spend so much money, because we can add cheese, ham, paprika, and onion to our omelet, and it is perfect for people who have a very rushed life, as it not only gives us a good amount of energy to do all our activities but also allows us not to waste much time in the kitchen.

Now, the ingredients of the omelet that we are going to recommend are the following:

- Six eggs.

- Two tablespoons of sour cream, or can also be whipped cream, to taste of the consumer.
- Salt to taste.
- Pepper to taste.
- Three ounces of grated cheese, no matter the type of cheese, can be smoked, gouda, the important thing is that it contains fat.
- Two ounces of butter.
- Five ounces of smoked ham cut into squares.
- Half medium onion, chopped into very small squares.
- Half green bell pepper, which has to be chopped into very thin strips.

It should be noted that you can add the ingredient you want, in addition to the proportions that were supplied here, are an estimate, you can add more or less to it.

After having the ingredients ready, we can proceed to the preparation of our recipe, in the following steps:

- Pour the six eggs and the cream over a bowl, then mix until you have a homogeneous and creamy mixture.
- Add salt and pepper.
- Add half of the grated cheese, after this, proceed to beat the mixture well again.
- Then, in a frying pan, melt the butter over medium heat, it is important that it is at this heat so that the butter does not burn.
- Pour the ham over the pan when the butter is melted, and proceed to fry the ham, paprika, and onions for a while, or until the onions are golden brown.
- Pour the eggs and cream mixture into the frying pan where the ham and onion were, then fry until the omelet is cooked.
- Reduce the heat for a while, and pour the rest of the grated cheese over the omelet, waiting for it to melt.
- Fold it.
- Take it out of the frying pan and cut it in half.

As you can see, the recipe is extremely simple. The same does not consume much time, less than ten minutes for sure, therefore, this recipe is very productive for people who have a very fast life, thus achieving a healthy and complete breakfast in less than ten minutes.

SCRAMBLED EGGS WITH FETA CHEESE

This is an extremely simple recipe, which allows people who do not have much experience cooking, to eat very healthy, very nutritious, and very rich in a short time, since the time it should take you to make this recipe is about ten or fifteen minutes. In addition to this, scrambled eggs can be added to any type of ingredients you want, such as bacon, ham, or even spinach. The ingredients for our recipe are as follows:

- Four eggs.
- Two good tablespoons of whipped cream, thick.
- Two tablespoons of butter.
- Four ounces of spinach.
- A finely chopped garlic clove.
- A quarter of shredded feta cheese.
- Salt to taste.
- Pepper to taste.
- Four ounces of bacon.

After we have all the ingredients ready, we can proceed to start with the preparation.

1. In a bowl, beat the eggs and cream until they are homogeneous and well creamy.
2. Cook the bacon until well cooked.
3. In a frying pan, melt the butter over medium heat.
4. After the butter is melted, proceed to add the other ingredients, such as spinach and garlic, wait until the spinach is cooked, you will notice if the spinach is withered.
5. Add the bacon to the pan, and add salt and pepper to taste.

6.   Pour over the frying pan, the mixture that contains the eggs, then wait until the edges of the frying pan begin to bubble, at this time, with the help of a spoon, stir from outside to inside, repeating the process until they are cooked.

7.   Remove the scrambled eggs from the pan, and add the feta cheese, in this part, you can also add a little more bacon if you choose.

As you can see, this recipe is extremely simple, so you can do it many times, you can change it and have different breakfasts for your whole week, just pretend you are the chef.

SNACKS

These foods are important when you've already eaten, but gives you a little hunger, for that reason, people turn to snacks, but in the case of those who do not have a ketogenic diet, they can go to some Cheetos or Doritos, but in our case, that we are with another type of food, we will have our nutritious snacks.

CHEESE CHIPS

This recipe is extremely simple, and you don't need many ingredients to make them since all you need is cheese and paprika.

The ingredients are exactly as follows:

*   Eight ounces of cheese, whether yellow, gouda, cheddar, provolone.
*   Half a spoonful of paprika.

As we can see, the ingredients are more than basic, to have our fantastic snack. The preparation is as follows.

1.   Preheat oven to 400°F.

2.   Grate the cheese of your preference, and place it in small piles on a tray to put it in the oven, it is important to say that the tray must be lined with parchment paper. It is important to leave enough space so that when they melt, the piles of cheese do not touch.

3.   Sprinkle the paprika over the grated cheese.

4.   Bake for about ten to eight minutes until you see that the cheese is ready, do not let the cheese burn.

5.   Let them cool and serve.

As you can see, this snack is extremely simple, and you don't need many ingredients, and so are the great majority of the snacks in the ketogenic diet. Therefore, we don't tell you more and go to the kitchen to see how delicious this recipe is.

CHAPTER 16:

LUNCH AND DINNER RECIPES

These other foods continue to be vital to our organism, to the point that we consider them to have the same importance as breakfast.

LUNCHES

After breakfast, between the twelve noon (12:00 pm) and the one o'clock (1:00 pm), we proceed to eat this meal, so that it continues to give us energy for the rest of the day.

KETO TACOS

This recipe is very simple since we are supplanting the carbohydrates of the cookie of the tacos, with cheese, which is an amazing idea and simple to make.

The ingredients are as follows:
- Two cups of cheddar cheese, gouda, grated parmesan.
- A spoonful of extra virgin olive oil.
- An onion chopped in small squares.
- Three cloves of garlic finely chopped.
- A pound of ground beef.
- Half a spoonful of ground cumin.
- Half a spoonful of paprika.
- Salt to taste.
- Black pepper to taste.
- Sour cream.
- Avocados, chopped in small squares.
- Fresh cilantro.

- Freshly chopped tomatoes, in small squares.

The next steps are as follows:

1. Preheat the oven to 400°F, and line the baking tray with the parchment paper.
2. Serve the cheese on the tray as piles, and make sure they have some distance so that when melted, the piles of cheese do not stick.
3. Bake until the cheese bubbles and begins to brown.
4. Let cool for about six minutes.
5. Then grease a muffin mold, then put the melted cheese over the muffin holes in the bottom. Try to give the cheese the shape of the mold.
6. In a saucepan over medium heat, melt butter and add onions, stirring until golden and tender, then add garlic.
7. Pour the ground meat over the frying pan with the onion and the garlic, with the help of a wooden spoon, stir the meat to cook it, it will be ready when it is no longer pink. Proceed to remove excess fat.
8. Sprinkle the paprika, cumin, red pepper, salt, and pepper over the meat.
9. On the cheese baskets that you already cooked, pour the meat, stuffing it with meat, avocado, tomato, and sour cream.

BOMB BURGERS

This is a very simple recipe, which will allow you to savor the deliciousness of the meat, no need to leave the diet.

The ingredients are as follows:

- Butter or cooking spray. To add it to the muffin mold.
- One pound of ground beef.
- Half a spoonful of garlic powder, if you like, you can add more.
- Salt to taste.
- Pepper to taste.
- Two tablespoons of butter, divided into twenty pieces.
- Eight ounces of cheddar cheese, divided into twenty pieces.

- Leaves lettuce well washed.
- Tomatoes in thin slices.
- Mustard.

The preparation process is very simple:

1. Preheat oven to about 400°F.
2. The muffin mold, you can add the cooking spray, or butter, so that what we are going to put there does not get stuck.
3. Season the meat with the garlic powder, salt, and pepper.
4. Take a tablespoon of meat, and put it in the muffin molds, then press it into the bottom. Then place a piece of butter on top, and press again, in order to completely cover the bottom.
5. Place a piece of cheese on top of the meat and butter, in each muffin cup, obviously, and then press the cheese, so that it is completely covered by the meat.
6. Bake until the meat is well cooked.
7. Remove the meat from each cup of muffin, do it carefully, it is recommended to use a spatula.
8. Serve the meat with the lettuce, tomato, and mustard.

As you may have seen, these recipes for a healthy lunch are very simple and quick to make, you don't need to be a chef to be able to cook this, so you don't need so much knowledge to be able to make our lunches.

DINNERS

This is the last meal of our day; for this reason, this takes on a fundamental importance, and that is why it is important to make a good dinner.

BROCCOLI KETO SALAD

This is a very simple recipe, which will allow you to have a diet that will provide you with good nutrition and helps you to continue with your ketosis process.

The ingredients are as follows:

- Salt to taste.
- Three broccoli, chopped into small pieces.
- Half a cup of grated yellow cheddar cheese.
- A quarter onion, cut into very thin slices.
- One-quarter cup sliced toasted almonds.
- Three slices of bacon, well cooked and toasted, which you can place as you like in your salad, either shredded or chopped.
- Two spoonfuls of chives, fresh and freshly chopped.
- Two-thirds of a cup of mayonnaise.
- Three spoonfuls of cider vinegar.
- One tablespoon of Dijon mustard.
- Freshly ground black pepper.

The steps to cook our broccoli salad are as follows:

1. Boil a considerable amount of water in a pot, about six cups of water.
2. Prepare a large bowl of ice water.
3. Pour the broccoli over the pot of boiling water, cook until tender; this may take an interval of one or two minutes.
4. Remove and place in a bowl of ice water until cool.
5. Drain the broccoli flowers with a sieve.
6. In another bowl, place the mayonnaise, vinegar, mustard, pepper, and salt, and beat everything to combine the ingredients of the dressing, you must achieve a homogeneous mixture.
7. In the bowl where you are going to serve the salad, pour the broccoli, grated cheddar cheese, onion, toasted almonds, and bacon, stir and then pour over them the dressing, mix until all the ingredients are covered by the dressing.
8. Refrigerate until ready to serve.

As you could see, the recipe has no major complication and can be done in less than an hour, you don't need so much knowledge to make the salad, and you are feeding us very well.

CHICKEN WITH BACON, CHEESE AND RANCH DRESSING

This recipe is very simple, and very tasty, because who doesn't like chicken, or bacon, or melted cheese?. Well, this recipe brings the three things together, a perfect combination and full of flavor.

The ingredients are as follows:
- Four slices of thick bacon, a little wide.
- Four boneless chicken breasts. It's important that you don't have skin or anything, you could also use chicken Milanese.
- Salt to taste.
- Pepper to taste.
- Two spoonfuls of ranchero seasoning.
- A cup and a half of grated mozzarella cheese, you can also eat it with cheddar cheese, to give a more "American" touch.
- Chopped chives.

As you can see in the ingredients, nothing from the other world is asked for; we could even say that it is usual. Therefore, the preparation of this recipe does not come out very expensive, and besides, it does not consume much time, as you will see below:

1. In a frying pan over medium heat, proceed to cook the bacon, leaving them to fry on their own fat and leaving them crispy, turning them from time to time. This can last about eight minutes. It's best to do all of this on a large pan.
2. After the bacon is cooked, remove it to a plate and drain the remaining fat from each bacon, we recommend lining it with kitchen paper.
3. Drain the frying pan a little, throwing away a little of the fat that the bacon has thrown away, but we will not throw away all of it, but we will leave two or three spoonfuls of bacon oil.

4. Season your chicken with salt and pepper to taste.

5. Return the pan to medium heat, a little higher now, and proceed to put the chicken pieces, cook until the chicken is golden and ready, so that it is not raw, this can take about six minutes.

6. Lower the heat of your pan, and then add the powder or ranch dressing to the chicken, and finally, coat it with mozzarella or cheddar cheese.

7. Cover the frying pan with its lid, and wait for the cheese to melt, and bubbles begin to bubble out of it.

8. Chop the bacon in small pieces, and proceed to pour it over the cheese, do the same with the spring onion.

As you could see, this recipe is extremely simple and very tasty, as are most recipes that have a ketogenic food base. Therefore, we only have to tell you to keep practicing and make many more recipes to see that having this way of eating is not boring quite the opposite.

CHAPTER 17:
DRINKS AND DESSERTS

A positive aspect of the keto diet is the fact that we can continue to eat deliciously without so many limitations as our body goes into ketosis, cravings or that feeling of anxiety will disappear.

However, it is common that we have a craving from time to time and much more if before changing our eating habits we had the habit of eating sweets in large quantities, keto desserts will be our salvation and we can enjoy a good snack that satisfies our cravings without going out of line.

It has always been believed that healthy eating is a drastic and limiting change in our lives, and even has the belief that a snack has to be a fruit; if we look at this case, most of these fruits do not favor the keto diet, so we should look for other healthy alternatives that can help us.

Next, we will show you different types of desserts that we can make in the keto diet:

Keto Recipes That Do Dot Need to Be Cooked in the Oven

PEANUT BUTTER LINT FAT BOMBS

It is known that peanut butter is a delight if we add chocolate is a bomb explosion of flavors.

Ingredients:
- 1 cup of whipped cream
- 3 tablespoons natural peanut butter
- 100 grams of cream cheese
- 1 tablespoon vanilla
- 50 grams unsweetened chocolate (preferably dark chocolate)

Preparation mode:

1. In a bowl, add the whipped cream and stir until doubled in size.

2. In a separate bowl, mix the cream cheese with the natural peanut butter, chocolate, and vanilla; and mix until it looks like a soft, creamy lint.

3. Then we are going to unite all the ingredients in the same bowl, and we will be mixing slowly until they integrate correctly and are soft.

4. Additionally, we can add grated chocolate to decorate.

The best part is that this recipe only takes:

➢ Net carbohydrates: 2 g

➢ Calories: 140 g

➢ Fat: 14 g

➢ Proteins: 3 g

KETO CHEESECAKE

Ingredients:

- 120 g. cream cheese
- ¼ cup of sweetener
- ¼ cup thick whipped cream
- 2 tablespoons sour cream
- 60 grams of unsweetened pastry chocolate
- ½ cup whipped cream

Preparation:

1. With the help of a mixer, mix the cream cheese, sour cream, whipped cream, and sweetener.

2. Fill a cupcake mold with the mixture.

3. We take the refrigerator for 3 hours or the freezer for an hour and a half.

4. For the ganache:

5. Melt the chocolate pastry in the microwave.

6. Add the thick cream to whip.

7.   Mix gently until it compacts, or you get a thick consistency.

8.   Decorate to taste.

With this delicious recipe, we are enjoying a delicious combination of flavors without losing our line that has only:

➢ Carbohydrates: 3 g.

➢ Calories: 300 g.

➢ Fats: 35 g.

➢ Proteins: 5 g.

COCONUT BISCUITS

With Only 3 Ingredients (not baked)

- 3 cups finely grated coconut flakes.
- 1 cup coconut oil
- ½ cup of sweetener

Preparation:

1.   In a bowl, mix the ingredients until we obtain a manipulable dough.

2.   Form uniform balls and crush them into the shape of a biscuit.

3.   Place each cookie 1 finger away in a tray with parchment paper.

4.   Refrigerate until firm

This delicious recipe can be kept covered at room temperature for 7 days. If you only have the mixture, you can freeze it for up to 2 months.

Keto Recipes That Need an Oven for Preparation

CHOCOLATE CAKE OR KETOLATE CAKE

Ingredients:

For the cake:

- 1 1/2 cup almond flour

- 2/3 Tbsp sugar-free cocoa powder
- 3/4 cup coconut flour
- 2 tbsp. baking powder
- 2 tbsp. baking soda
- 500 grams of butter
- 1 cup sweetener
- 4 eggs
- 1 tablespoon vanilla
- 1 cup almond milk
- 1/3 cup of coffee

For frosting:

- 60 grams of cream cheese
- 250 grams of butter
- ½ cup sweetener (or to taste)
- 1/2 tbsp sugar-free cocoa powder
- 1/2 tbsp coconut flour
- 3/4 cup whipping cream

Preparation:

1. Preheat oven to 350 °.
2. Grease the mold where the cake is going to be baked.
3. In a large bowl, combine all dry ingredients
4. With the help of a blender, mix all the liquid ingredients.
5. Combine ingredients in one bowl
6. Bake for 30 minutes.
7. Preparation of the glaze: In a large bowl, with the help of a mixer mix the cream cheese and butter until a smooth mixture is formed, then gradually add the rest of the ingredients.
8. Decorate and serve

CHOCOLATE CHIP COOKIES

Ingredients:

- 2 eggs
- 250 grams melted butter
- 2 tablespoons whipping cream
- 2 teaspoons of vanilla
- 2 3/4 cup almond flour
- 1/4 cup granulated sugar keto-friendly
- 100 grams of dark chocolate in drops.

Preparation:

1. Preheat oven to 350 °.
2. In a large bowl mix the egg and butter
3. Then add the waiting cream and vanilla and mix until you add the dry ingredients.
4. Finally, add the chocolate sparks.
5. Form uniform balls and in a tray with parchment paper, place them with three fingers apart.
6. Bake for 15 minutes

What Beverages Other Than Water Can I Drink on the Keto Diet?

Among the most prominent are:

- Water infusions
- Hot or cold coffee
- Hot or cold tea
- Diet Sodas
- Smoothies keto

How to make Keto Infusions?

To make infusions is simpler than you can imagine. Besides that, they are very healthy giving us the capacity of up to 4 liters for preparation.

Strawberry and Cucumber Infusion

Ingredients:

- 500 g strawberries
- Cucumber slices
- 2 liters of water

OTHER TYPES OF KETO DRINKS

HOT CHOCOLATE

Ingredients:

- 2 spoonfuls. cocoa powder without sugar
- 2 1/2 teaspoons sweetener
- 1 1/4 cup water
- 1/4 cup heavy cream
- 1/4 teaspoon vanilla
- Whipped cream to taste, to decorate

Preparation:

1. In a saucepan, mix the cocoa, sweetener, and water on a medium-low heat until it dissolves correctly.
2. Increase heat to medium and add remaining ingredients, stirring constantly.
3. When it is hot enough, add the vanilla and serve in a cup.

KETO SMOOTHIE

Ingredients:

- Spinach
- coconut milk
- whey protein,
- Almonds

- Sweet potato starch
- psyllium seeds

Preparation:

Beat all ingredients in blender and serve.

STRAWBERRY MILKSHAKE

- 1 cup fresh strawberries
- 1 tsp vanilla
- 1 tbsp. coconut or almond oil
- 450ml coconut milk or Greek yogurt

Preparation:

Beat all ingredients in blender and serve.

CHIA SHAKE

Ingredients:

- 1 tablespoon of chia seeds (previously soaked in water for 10 minutes)
- ¼ cup coconut milk
- 1 avocado
- 1 tsp. cocoa beans
- 1 tsp. cocoa powder
- 1 tablespoon protein powder
- 1 tbsp. coconut oil

Preparation:

We blend all the ingredients so that all the ingredients are mixed correctly if you feel that it has become thick, you can add a little water.

Serve and enjoy

KETO GREEN MILKSHAKE

Ingredients:

- Cucumber
- Pineapple
- Kiwi
- Ginger
- Parsley
- 2 cups of water

Preparation:

Mix all the ingredients in a blender and serve.

Can I drink alcohol if I'm on the Keto Diet?

If we ingest alcohol while following the keto diet, our body will use this as a way to get energy before using the fat, but this could be contradictory because in the state of ketosis we look for our body to burn fat to get energy and thus lose weight, so the intake of alcohol could achieve effects contrary to those we seek to get.

CHAPTER 18:

QUICK AND EASY DIFFERENT RECIPES

We know that time is money, but it still doesn't mean that just because we have a tight schedule in our daily routine, we can't afford to eat healthy. Below we will show you recipes for healthy and delicious foods that you can prepare in less than 20 minutes.

QUICK SALAD

Ingredients:

- 40 grams of green leaves (Lettuce or so)
- ½ sliced spring onion
- 1 carrot
- 1/2 avocado
- 20 gr. paprika
- 20 gr. tomatoes
- 120 grams of smoked salmon or chicken
- ¼ cup olive oil

Preparation:

1. First, we will chop all our ingredients to our preference
2. In a medium jar (or our taste) we will serve the green leaves at the bottom, followed by this we will add the rest of the ingredients, finally add the salmon or chicken and olive oil.
3. This way, we will have a quick and delicious lunch.

MUSHROOM TORTILLA

Ingredients:

- 4 eggs

- 25 g. butter
- 50 g. Grated cheese
- ¼ chopped yellow onion
- 4 mushrooms, sliced
- salt and pepper

Preparation:

1. In a bowl, mix the eggs with a fork until foamy, then add salt and pepper to taste.
2. In a frying pan over medium heat, fry the mushrooms together with the onion and butter until they are cooked.
3. Add the egg to the frying pan.
4. When the tortilla is half cooked, add the cheese
5. Using a spatula, fold the tortilla in half to give it consistency.
6. Remove from frying pan and serve.

SMOKED SALMON AND AVOCADO MEAL

Ingredients:

- 250 g smoked salmon
- 2 avocados
- salt and pepper

Preparation:

1. Chop the avocado into strips and place on a plate.
2. Serve the lounge
3. Add salt and pepper to taste.

CRISPY BACON

Ingredients

- 400 g bacon

- 1 cauliflower
- 50 grams of butter
- salt and pepper
- Oil

Preparation:

1. Chop the cauliflower into small pieces
2. Chop bacon into small pieces
3. Fry in a frying pan with butter until golden brown and crisp.
4. Serve with salt and pepper to taste.

CRABMEAT AND EGG

Ingredients

- 3 eggs
- 500 g canned crab meat
- 2 avocados
- ½ cup mayonnaise
- 1½ oz. spinach
- 2 tablespoons olive oil
- salt and pepper

Preparation:

1. we boil the eggs for about 10 minutes
2. We season the crab meat to your preference
3. Once the eggs are boiled, we'll remove the shell.
4. Serve on a plate with avocado chopped in strips
5. mix the mayonnaise with the crab meat
6. We'll sprinkle olive oil for seasoning.

CONCLUSION

Thank you for making it through to the end of Keto and intermittent fasting: Your Essential Guide for a Low-Carb diet to perfect mind-body balance, weight loss, with ketogenic Recipes to Maximize Your Health, we really hope it was informative and that you were able to learn all of the tools you needed to achieve your goal with the keto diet, whatever it was.

If you are reading this, it is because you made it through the book. And because of that, we want to congratulate you, since it means that you are completely decided and moving forward to change your body, your lifestyle, and most importantly, your mental and physical health. We really know that making such a change is not an easy task, and that is why we are really happy that you are so decided and interested in this diet.

Since the moment you bought this book, you became a winner. You became a champion. Not everyone is brave enough to dare to change in such a drastic way their nutrition and their feeding methods. Most people fear to fail, but what differences the normal people from the special people, the people that success, the people that get out of the comfort zone, is the discipline and perseverance towards reaching their goals.

Even if you are starting and find it really hard, or if you started but quitted, don't give up, keep pushing, keep trying and see amazing and unbelievable changes to start happening. This does not only applies to this diet but for everything in the life.

Finally, if you found this book useful in any way, a review on Amazon is always appreciated!

Keto Chaffle Cookbook

An Easy Guide to Make Delicious Chaffles with Low Carb Recipes to Lose Weight, Improve Your Health and Satisfy your soul. With Pictures!

By

Zoe Nelson

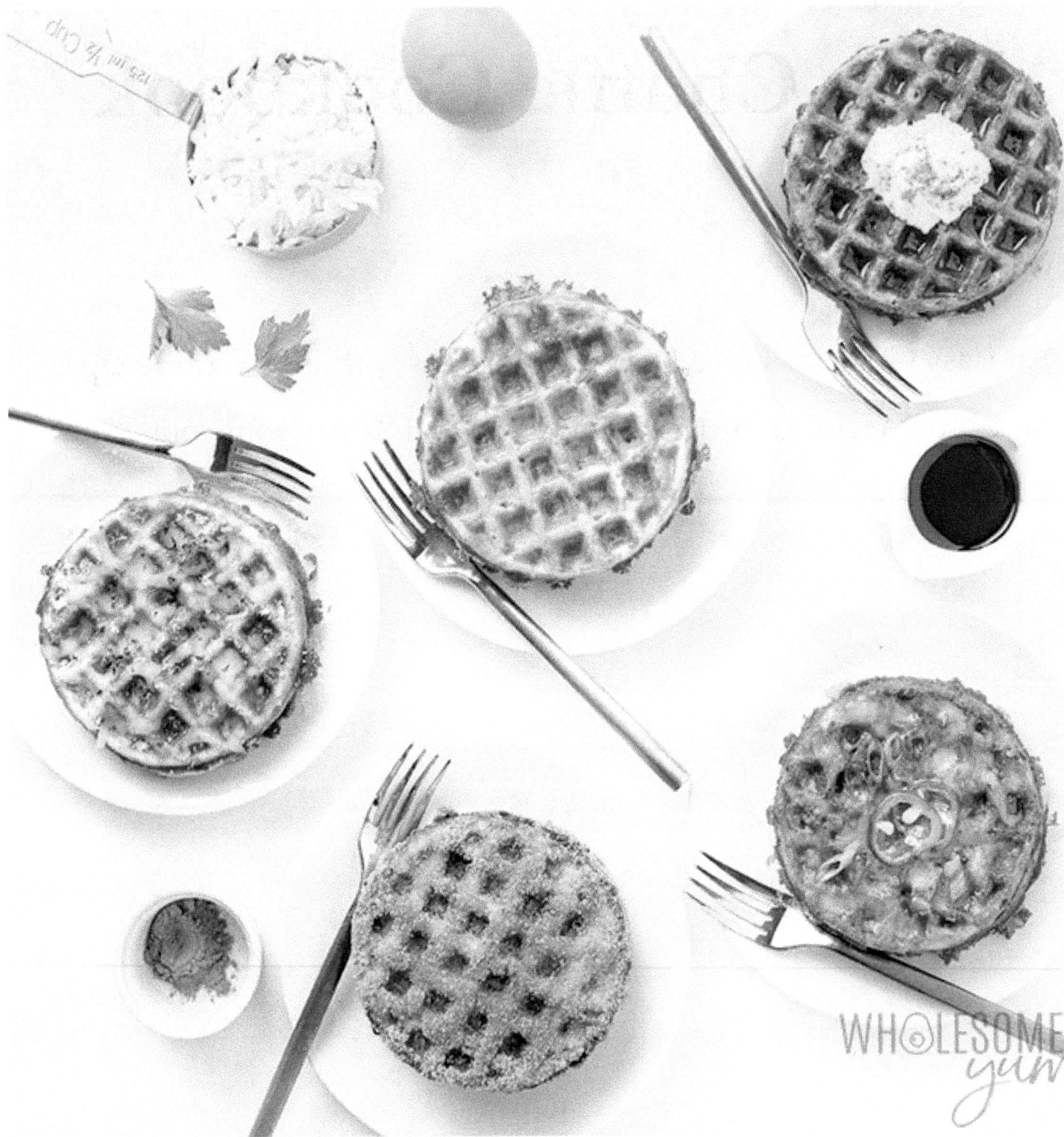

INTRODUCTION

Ketogenic refers to a low-carbohydrate diet. The aim is to eat more calories from fat and protein while eating fewer calories from carbohydrates. The carbohydrates that are easiest to digest, such as starch, pastries, soda, and white bread, are the first to go. When you consume fewer than 50 g of carbohydrates a day, your body easily runs out of energy. This normally takes three or four days. Then you'll begin to break down fat and protein for energy, potentially resulting in weight loss. Ketosis is the term for this state. It's crucial to remember that the ketogenic diet is a short-term diet designed to help you lose weight rather than change your lifestyle. A ketogenic diet is more often used to reduce weight, although it may also be used to treat medical problems such as epilepsy. It can even benefit those suffering from heart failure, some brain disorders, and even acne, although further study is required. Since the keto diet contains too much fat, adherents must ingest fat at every meal time. In a normal 2K-calorie diet, that would seem like 165 g of fat, 40 g of carbohydrates, and 75 g of protein. The exact ratio, on the other hand, is determined by your basic requirements. Nuts (walnuts, almonds), avocados, seeds, olive oil and tofu are among the healthier unsaturated fats allowed on the keto diet. However, oils (coconut, palm), butter, lard, and peanut butter all contain high amounts of saturated fats. Protein is an essential aspect of the keto diet, although it is also difficult to discern between protein items that are lean and protein products rich in fat(saturated), such as beef, bacon, and pork. What for fruits and vegetables? While fruits are generally rich in carbohydrates, unique fruits may be obtained in limited quantities (generally berries) Leafy greens (like kale, chard, Swiss chard, and spinach), broccoli, cauliflower, asparagus, tomatoes, brussels sprouts, bell peppers, garlic, cucumbers, mushrooms, summer squashes, as well as celery are also rich in carbohydrates. One cup of sliced broccoli includes about six carbohydrates. At the same time, there are several possible keto hazards, such as liver deficiency, liver complications, constipation, kidney disorders, and so on. As a result, we can also keep our Keto diet portions in check.

UNDERSTANDING THE KETOGENIC DIET

This chapter delves into the Ketogenic diet in depth. The chapter further discusses which foods to consume on the Keto diet and which foods to stop while on this diet. The Keto diet is often explained in-depth, including how it functions and what health advantages it provides.

The ketogenic diet (or keto diet) is a high-fat, low-carbohydrate diet with various health benefits. Evidently, more than 20 studies suggest that this form of diet will help you lose weight and boost your wellbeing. Diabetes patients, epilepsy patients, patients suffering from Alzheimer's disease, as well as cancer can all benefit from ketogenic diets.

1.1 WHAT IS KETO?

The ketogenic diet is a very low carbohydrate, high-fat diet that has a lot in common with the Atkins diet and other low-carb diets. It necessitates a significant reduction of carbohydrate consumption and a replacement with fat. This reduction of carbohydrates puts the body into a metabolic condition known as ketosis. As this occurs, the body's energy production of fat-burning skyrockets. In addition, it converts fat into ketones in the liver, which will supply energy to the brain. Ketogenic diets can result in substantial reductions in insulin as well as blood sugar levels. This, along with the increased ketones, has numerous health benefits.

Ketogenic Diets Come in Many Forms

There are a few variations of the ketogenic diet, including:

The traditional ketogenic diet consists of a diet that is low in carbs, mild in protein, and strong in fats. It usually has a 75 percent fat content, a 5% carbohydrate content, and a 20% protein content.

The cyclic ketogenic diet entails high-carb reefed cycles, such as five ketogenic days accompanied by two days of high carbohydrate use.

A ketogenic diet with particular goals: The diet requires carbs to be inserted in between exercises.

Protein-rich ketogenic diet: This is comparable to a normal keto diet, but it contains extra protein. Usually, the ratio is 60 percent fat, 5% sugars, and 35 percent protein.

However, only normal and protein-rich ketogenic diets have been extensively studied. More complex keto diets, such as targeted or cyclic keto, are mainly utilized by bodybuilders and athletes.

Ketogenic Diet Health Benefits

In fact, the keto diet first gained popularity as a means of treating neurological conditions, such as epilepsy. Following that, research has shown that diet can help with a broad variety of health issues:

Heart disease: The keto diet has been found to decrease risk factors such as body fat, blood sugar, HDL cholesterol and blood pressure.

Alzheimer's disease: The ketogenic diet can ease Alzheimer's symptoms while still delaying the disease's progression.

Epilepsy: Research has demonstrated that a ketogenic diet can significantly reduce seizures in children with epileptic seizures.

Cancer: The diet is actually being used to control a number of diseases and to delay tumor development.

Acne: Lower insulin levels, as well as less sugar or fried food diets, will aid acne recovery.

Parkinson's disease: According to one report, diet can help relieve the effects of Parkinson's disease.

Brain injuries: One study found that the diet would also increase concussions and improve recovery after a brain injury.

Polycystic ovary syndrome: A ketogenic diet may help lower insulin levels and can be helpful in the treatment of polycystic ovary syndrome.

What foods can you consume on a ketogenic diet?

The majority of your meals will revolve around the following foods:
- Salmon, mackerel and tuna are representations of fatty fish.
- Look for pastured eggs, whole eggs, or omega-3 eggs.
- Seek for grass-fed butter plus cream wherever possible.
- Red meat, ham, sausage, turkey, bacon, chicken and steak are all examples of meat.
- Non-processed cheese (goat, cheddar, mozzarella, blue, or cream).
- Flax seeds, walnuts, almonds, pumpkin seeds, chia seeds and other nuts and beans
- Avocado oil, olive oil and coconut oil are the other safe oils.
- Salt, spices and pepper, as well as a variety of herbs, may be used as condiments.
- Avocados: entire avocados or guacamole made freshly.
- Low-carb vegetables including greens, tomatoes, onions, peppers and other related veggies.

Foods to avoid on a ketogenic diet include:

Carbohydrate-rich diets can be avoided as much as possible.

The following is a selection of items that must be eliminated or reduced on a ketogenic diet:

- Sugary drink, ice cream, soda, smoothies, cake, candy and other sugary items
- Wheat, pasta, cereals, rice, and other wheat-based products are examples of starches or grains.
- Sweet potatoes, parsnips, parsnips, potatoes, carrots and other tubers & root vegetables
- Reduced-calorie or low-fat foods are extremely processed and abundant in carbohydrates.
- Fruit: All fruits, with the exception of tiny bits of berries like strawberries.
- Chickpeas, lentils, peas, kidney beans, and other legumes or beans
- Some sauces/condiments: They are also high in unhealthy fat and sugar.
- Unhealthy fats: Limit the intake to mayonnaise, processed vegetable oils, and other processed fats.
- Alcohol: Because of their carb content, certain alcoholic beverages will shake you out of ketosis.
- Dietary ingredients that are sugar-free: Alcohols, which are often rich in sugar, may influence ketone levels in certain situations. These objects seem to have passed through a lot of refining as well.

1.2 WHAT IS THE KETO DIET, AND HOW DOES IT WORK?

The "ketogenic" keto diet consists of consuming a moderate level of protein, a heavy amount of fat, and relatively little carbohydrates; also, the fruit is forbidden. As for every diet fad, the advantages to adherents include improved vitality, weight reduction, and mental clarity. Is the ketogenic diet, though, what it's cracked up to be?

Dietitians and nutritionists are quiet on the topic. Low-carb diets like keto appear to assist with weight loss in the short term, but they are no more successful than any other self-help or conventional diet. They still don't seem to be enhancing athletic results.

The ketogenic diet was created to treat epilepsy instead of losing weight. In the 1920s, physicians found that holding people on low-carb diets induced their bodies to use fat as the predominant fuel source rather than glucose. When only fat is available for the body to combust or burn, the body converts fats to fatty acids, which are then converted to ketones, which can be used and taken up to power the body's cells.

Currently, feeding the body exclusively ketones prevents epilepsy for unclear causes. However, with the advent of anti-seizure medicines, few patients with epilepsy rely on ketogenic diets anymore, while certain people who may not respond to medications may benefit. Low carb diets like the Atkins diet, which gained popularity in the early 2000s, also spawned keto diets for weight loss. In comparison, all groups of meatier-meal diets restrict carbohydrates. This diet does not have a set structure, although most routines provide for fewer than fifty grams of carbs per day.

A keto diet causes the body to enter a state known as ketosis, in which the body's cells become completely reliant on ketones for nutrition. It's not exactly clear that this leads to weight loss, but ketosis decreases appetite and can affect hunger-controlling hormones, including insulin. As a consequence, proteins and fats can keep humans fuller longer than sugars, resulting in lower net calorie intake.

In one head-to-head comparison, researchers looked at 48 separate diet trials in which subjects were randomly allocated to one of the well-known diets. Low-carb diets like South Beach, Atkins, and Zone, as well as low-fat diets like Ornish diets and portion restriction diets like Weight Watchers and Jenny Craig, were among the options.

Every diet resulted in greater weight loss than almost no diet after six months, according to the results. Low-carb and low-fat dieters lost almost equal amounts of weight as compared to non-dieters, with low-carb dieters losing 19 pounds on average versus low-fat dieters dropping 17.6 pounds (7.99 kilograms). At 12 months, both diet styles displayed symptoms of dropping off, with low-fat and low-carb dieters being 16 pounds (7.27 kg) smaller on average than non-dieters.

There were few differences in weight reduction within the diets of designated people. This is in line with the practice of recommending every diet that an individual practice in order to lose weight.

Another study of well-known diets discovered the Atkins diet, which results in greater weight loss than merely teaching people about portion control. Nevertheless, several of the scientific researched about this low-carb diet featured licensed dietitians assisting respondents in making food decisions, rather than the self-directed approach used by most people. This has been seen in other diet studies, according to the researchers, and the tests' results seem to be more positive in the real world than the weight loss.

Finally, a simple comparison between low-carb versus low-fat dieting revealed that there was a statistically significant difference in the amount of weight lost over a year. Low-carbohydrate dieters dropped an average of 13 pounds (6 kg), compared to 11.7 pounds for low-fat dieters (5.3 kg).

Ketogenic diets may help us lose weight, but they are no more successful than other diet methods. Since carbohydrate reserves in the body comprise water molecules, the bulk of the weight lost during the early stages of a ketogenic diet is water weight. This gives the scale an exciting amount at first, but weight reduction slows down with time.

What are the keto effects, and how can they help?

The advantages of a keto diet are close to that of other high-fat, low-carb diets, but it tends to be more successful than centrist low-carb diets. Keto is a low-carb, high-fat diet that maximizes health benefits. However, it will slightly raise the likelihood of complications.

Aid in weight loss

Weight reduction can be improved by converting the body into a fat-burning device. Insulin levels – the hormone that retains fat – are falling rapidly, suggesting that fat burning has risen dramatically. This seems to make it much easier to lose bodyweight without going hungry.

More than thirty high-quality observational studies show that low-carb and keto diets are more effective than other diets at losing weight.

Reverse type 2 diabetes by regulating blood sugar

A ketogenic diet has been shown in research to be successful in the treatment of type 2 diabetes, with total disease reversal occurring in certain instances. It makes perfect sense since keto removes the need for therapy, lowers blood sugar levels, and eliminates the potential negative consequences of high insulin levels.

Since a keto diet will reverse type 2 diabetes, it is likely to be helpful in preventing and reversing pre-diabetes. Keep in mind that "reversal" in this context refers to changing the disease, improving glucose tolerance, and reducing the need for care. It may be so drastically altered that after therapy, blood pressure returns to normal with time. In this context, reversal refers to progressing or deteriorating in the reverse direction of the condition. Changes in your lifestyle, on the other side, just succeed if you bring them into effect. If a person returns to the way of life he or she has before diabetes type 2 appeared and advanced, it is possible that success would return with time.

Improve your mental and physical performance:

Some people use ketogenic diets to boost their mental performance. It's also normal for people to feel more energized while they're in ketosis.

They don't need nutritional carbs for the brain on keto. It runs on ketones 24 hours a day, seven days a week, with a small amount of glucose synthesized in the liver. Carbohydrates are not necessary for the diet. As a result, ketosis leads to a steady flow of food (ketones) to the brain, avoiding significant blood sugar spikes. This will also assist with improved focus and attention, as well as clearing brain fog and improving mental awareness.

Epilepsy Treatment

The keto diet has been used to manage epilepsy since the 19th and 20th centuries and has proved to be effective. It has historically been used mainly for adolescents, although in recent years, it has also proved to be useful to adults. Or, used in conjunction with a keto diet, certain people with epilepsy might be able to take less to no anti-epileptic drugs while being seizure-free. This may help to reduce the drug's adverse effects while still improving cognitive capacity.

KETO CHAFFLE RECIPES

1 OREO CHAFFLES

(Ready in about 23 minutes | Serving 2 | Difficulty: Easy)

Per serving: Kcal 1381, Fat: 146g, Net Carbs: 14g, Protein: 17g

Ingredients

- 1/2 cup of Sugar-Free Chocolate Chips
- 1 tsp of Vanilla extract
- 3 Eggs
- 1/2 cup of butter
- 1/4 cup of sweetener

Cheese Frosting

- 4 ounces of Cream Cheese
- 4 ounces of butter
- 1/2 cup of Powdered Swerve
- 1 tsp of Vanilla extract
- 1/4 cup of Whipping Cream

Instructions

Melt chocolate and butter in a bowl in the microwave for around 1 minute. Stir to remove clumps. Mix vanilla, egg and sweetener in a bowl. Pour a quarter of the mixture into the waffle maker and cook for around 8 minutes. Mix frosting ingredients in the food processor's bowl in the meantime and make a smooth mixture. Spread frosting among two chaffles.

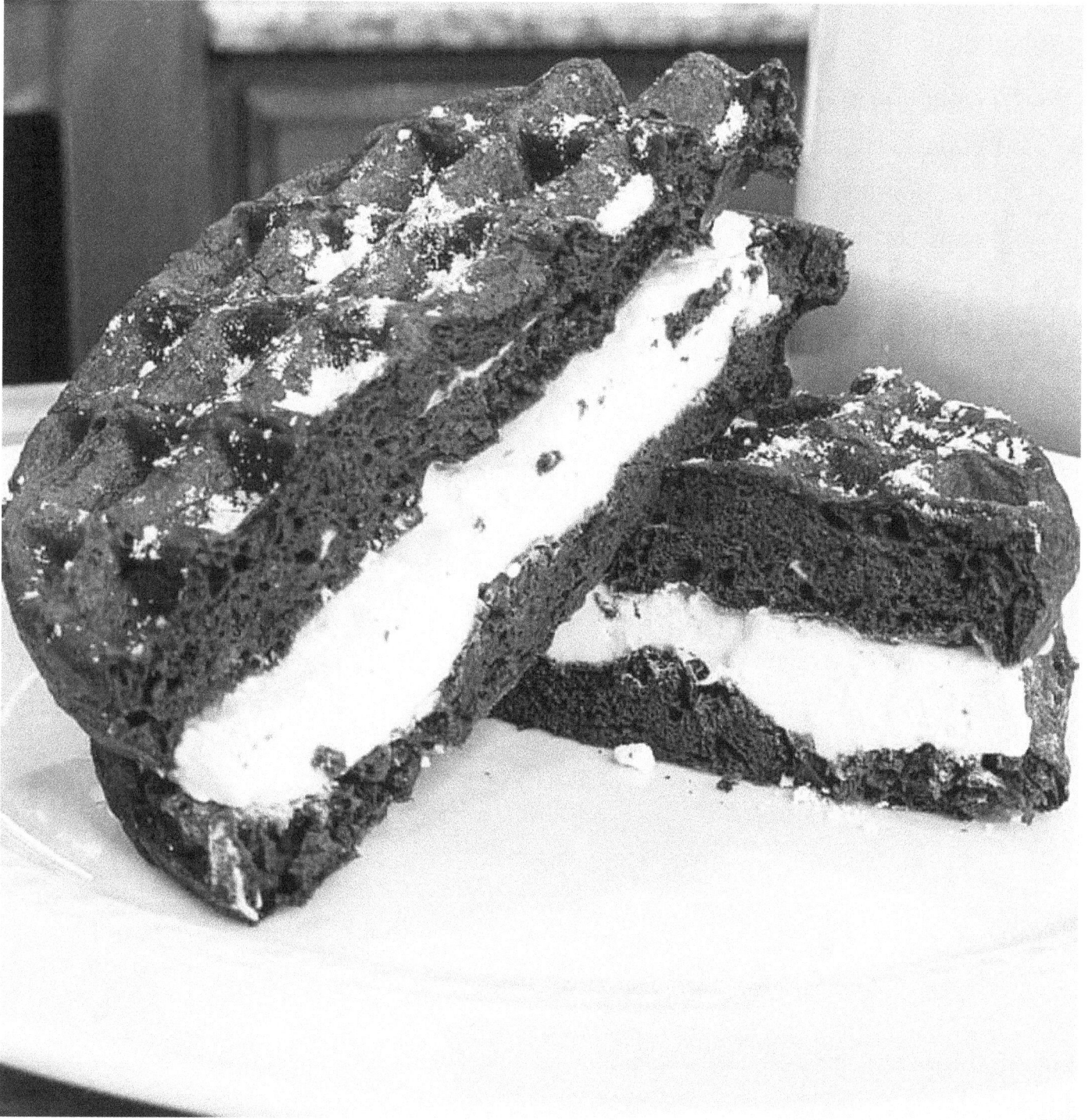

2 STRAWBERRY CHAFFLES

(Ready in about 35 minutes | Serving 8 | Difficulty: Moderate)

Per serving: Kcal 189, Fat: 14.3g, Net Carbs: 5.2g, Protein: 10g

Ingredients

- 3 oz of cream cheese
- 1 cup of whipped cream
- 2 beaten eggs
- 2 cups shredded mozzarella cheese
- 1/2 cup of almond flour
- 2 tsp of baking powder
- 3 tbsp of sweetener
- 8 strawberries
- 1 tbsp of sweetener

Instructions

Add mozzarella and cream cheese to a bowl and microwave for around 1 minute. Beat eggs and mix with baking powder, 3 tbsp sweetener and almond flour. Mix it with cheese and add to 2 diced strawberries. Place in the fridge for around 20 minutes. Dice the rest of the strawberries and add tbsp sweetener. Warm waffle iron and add the quarter mixture from the fridge to the center of the iron. Cook for around 7 minutes.

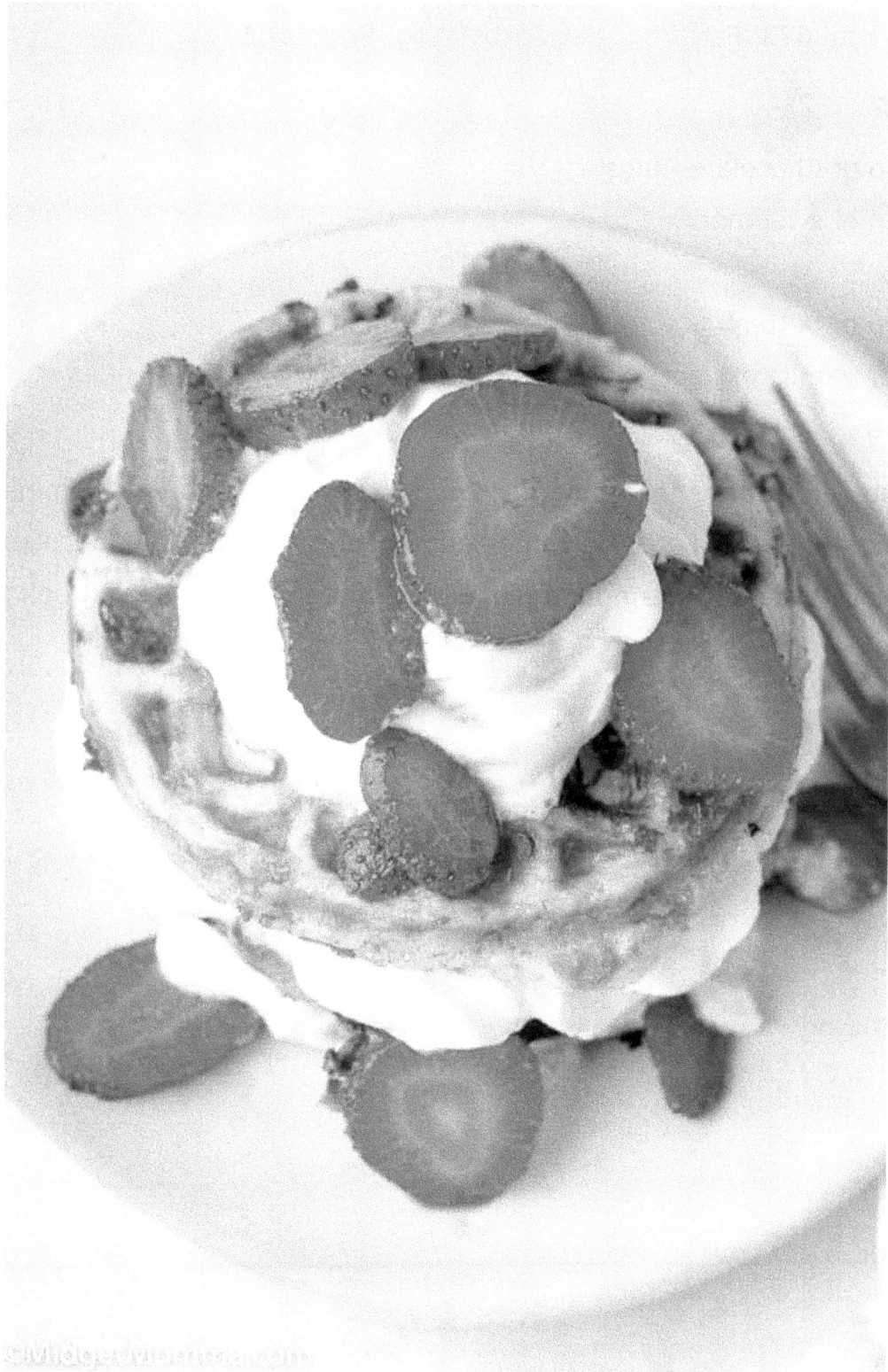

3 CHOCOLATE CHAFFLE

(Ready in about 18 minutes | Serving 2 | Difficulty: Easy)

Per serving: Kcal 672, Fat: 70g, Net Carbs: 11g, Protein: 13g

Ingredients

- 1/2 cup of Chocolate Chips
- 1/4 cup of sweetener
- 3 Eggs
- 1/2 cup of butter
- 1 tsp of Vanilla extract

Instructions

Melt chocolate and butter in a bowl in the microwave for around 1 minute. Stir and remove clumps. Blend sweetener, vanilla and eggs in a bowl. Add chocolate and butter and whisk. Pour the quarter amount of mixture into a waffle maker. Cook for around 8 minutes.

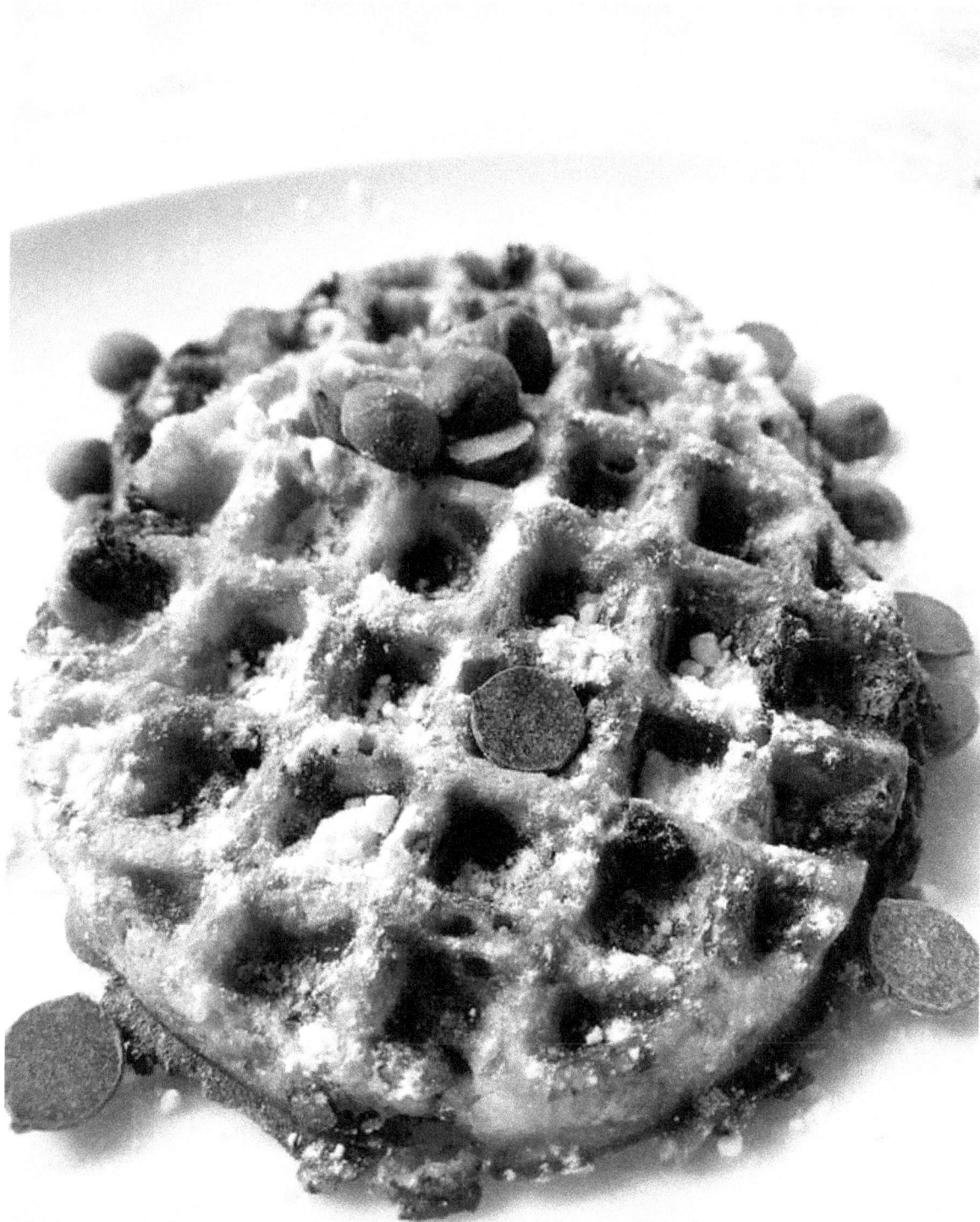

4 PUMPKIN CHAFFLES

(Ready in about 7 minutes | Serving 1 | Difficulty: Easy)

Per serving: Kcal 250, Fat: 15g, Net Carbs: 5g, Protein: 23g

Ingredients

- 1/2 cup mozzarella cheese shredded
- 1 1/2tbsp of pumpkin purée
- 1 beaten egg
- 1/2tsp of Swerve confectioners
- 1/4tsp of Pumpkin Pie Spice
- 1/2tsp of vanilla extract
- ⅛ tsp of maple extract

Instructions

Mix all the ingredients except mozzarella cheese in a bowl and mix. Add cheese and whisk. Spray waffle using cooking spray. Place half amount of batter in the center of the waffle maker. Cook for around 6 minutes. Repeat with the remaining batter.

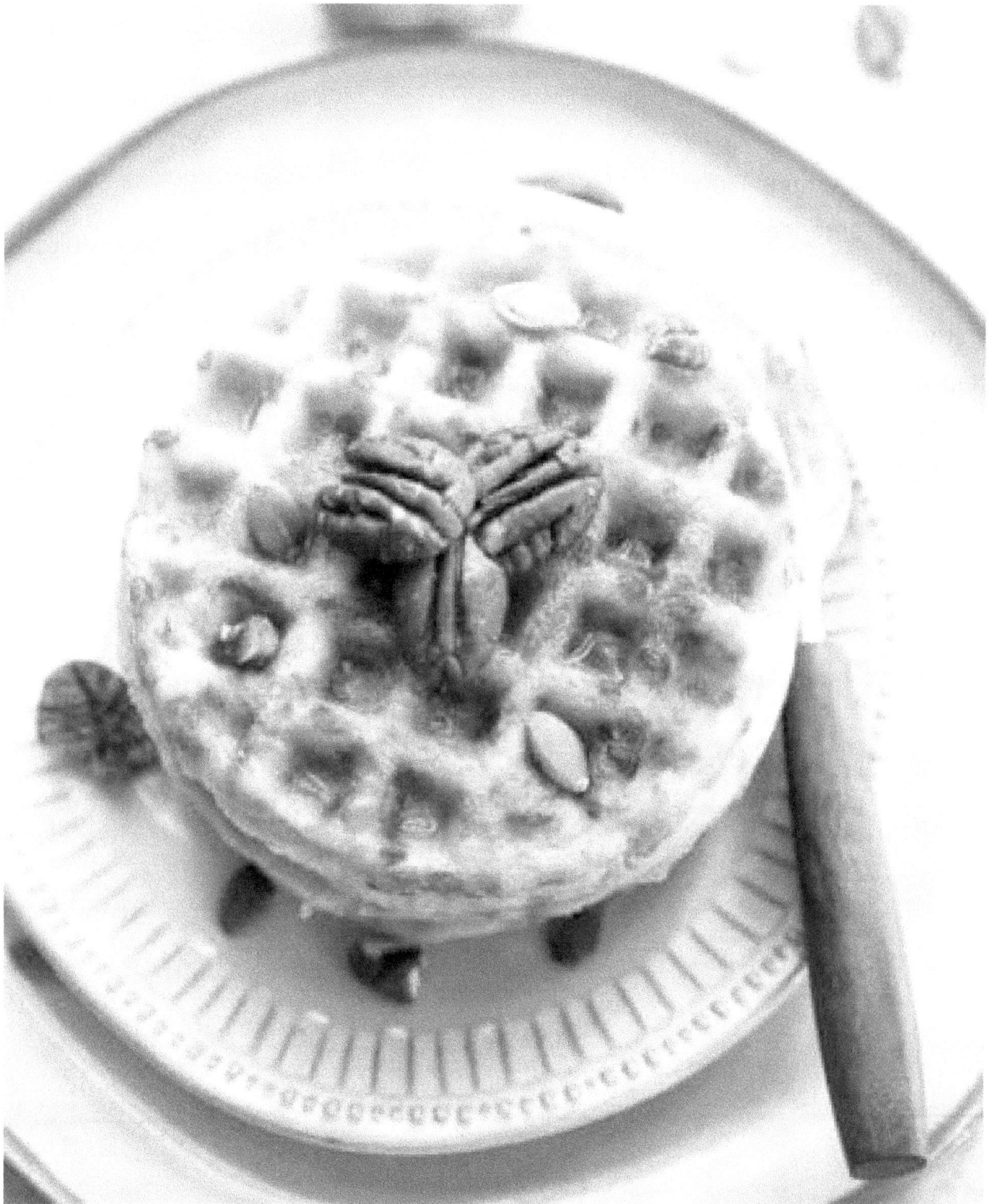

5 BASIC CHAFFLE

(Ready in about 8 minutes | Serving 2 | Difficulty: Easy)

Per serving: Kcal 208, Fat: 16g, Net Carbs: 4g, Protein: 11g

Ingredients

- 1 Big Egg
- 2 tbsp of Almond Flour
- 1/2 cup shredded Mozzarella cheese

Instructions

Preheat waffle iron for around 5 minutes. Microwave cheese for around 30 seconds. Add the rest of the ingredients and mix. Pour mixture that covers the surface of the waffle maker. Cook for around 4 minutes. Take out and place on a plate and repeat with the rest of the batter.

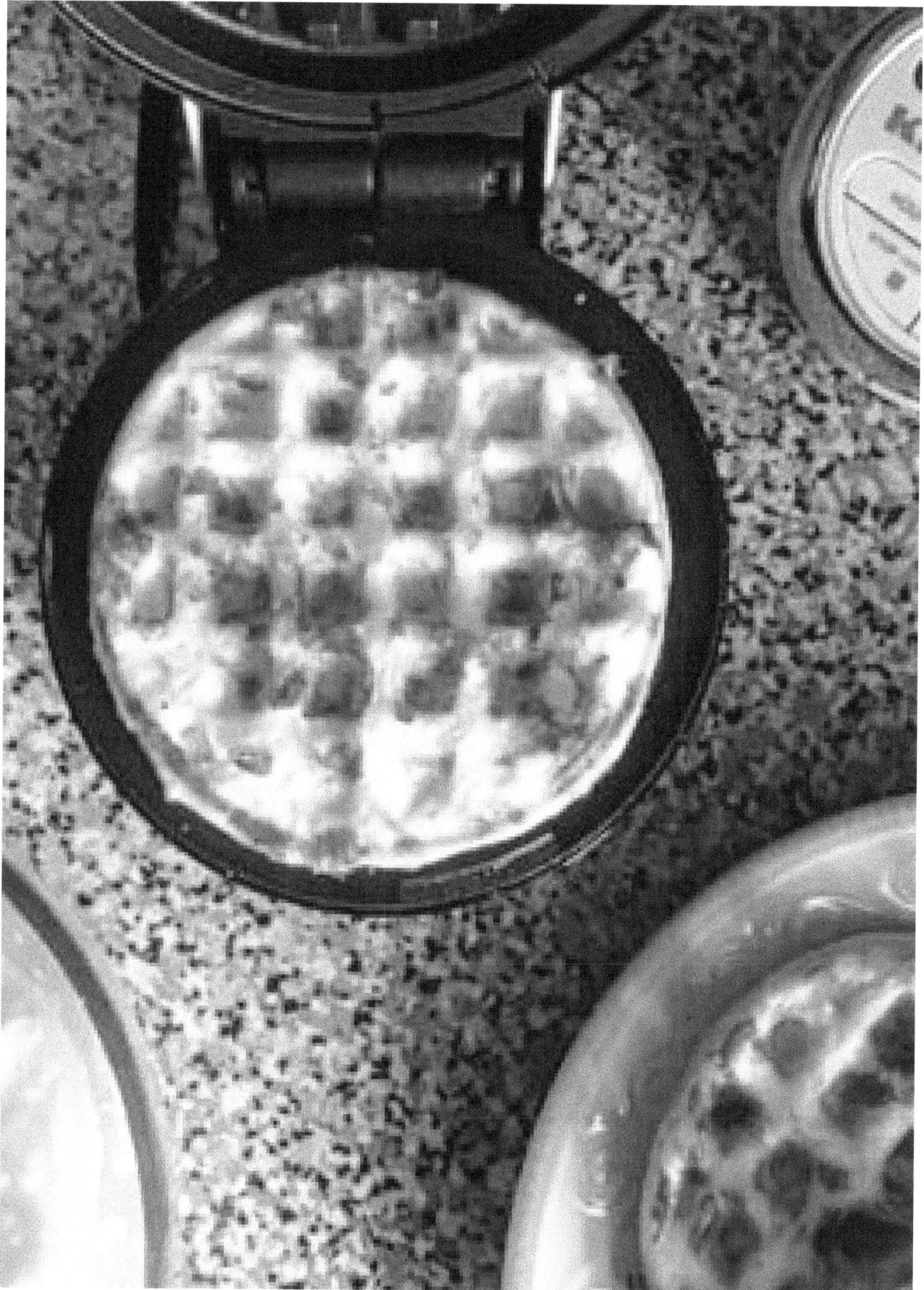

6 GARLIC CHAFFLES

(Ready in about 8 minutes | Serving 2 | Difficulty: Easy)

Per serving: Kcal 208, Fat: 16g, Net Carbs: 4g, Protein: 11g

Ingredients

- 1/3 cup Parmesan cheese Grated
- 1/2 cup shredded Mozzarella cheese
- 1 Big Egg
- 1/2 tsp of Italian seasoning
- 1 minced Garlic clove

Instructions

Preheat waffle iron for around 5 minutes. Microwave cream cheese for around 30 seconds. Add the rest of the ingredients except the toppings. Pour mixture that covers the surface of the waffle maker. Cook for around 4 minutes. Take out and place on a plate and repeat with the rest of the batter.

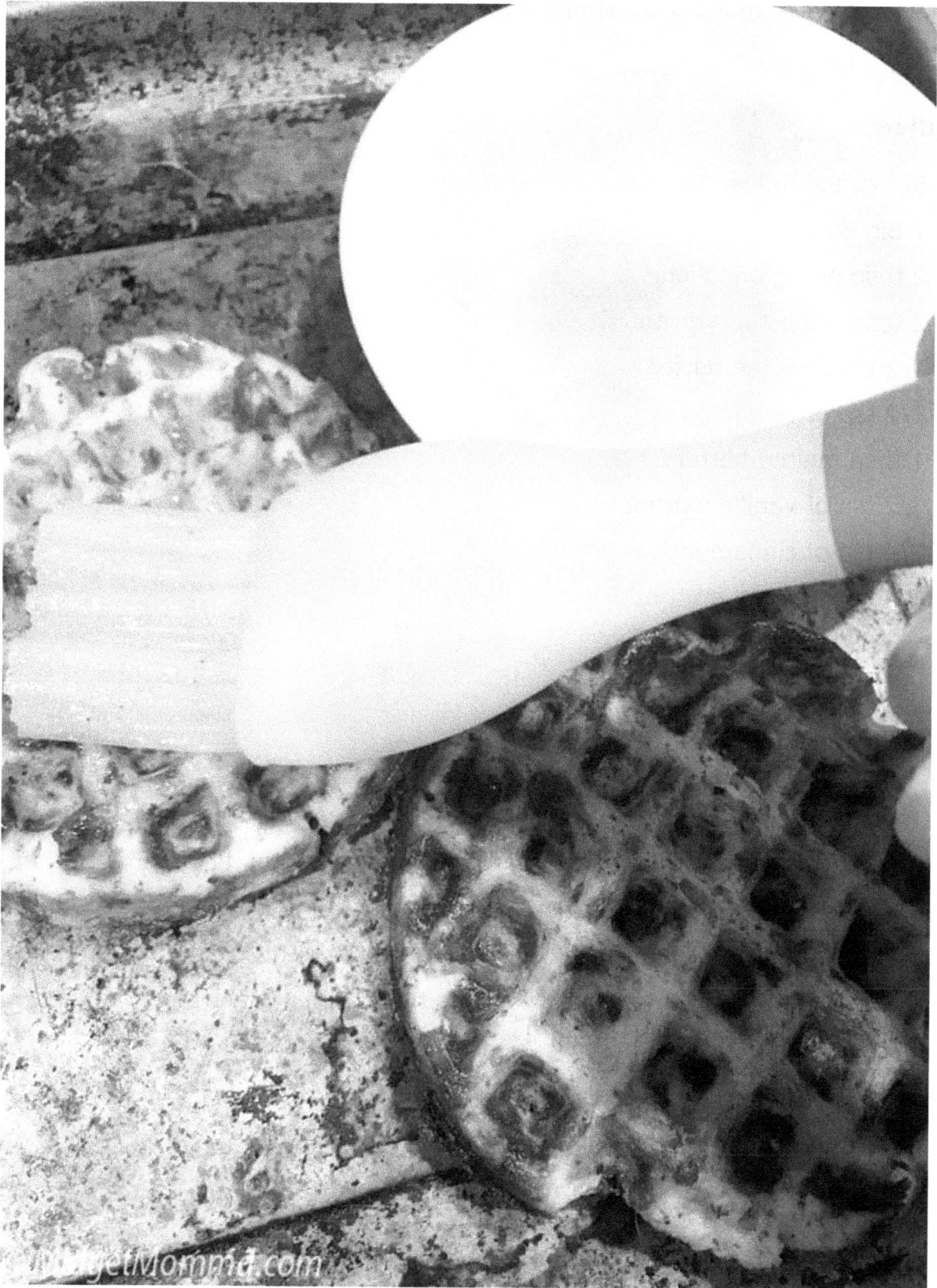

7 CINNAMON CHAFFLES

(Ready in about 8 minutes | Serving 2 | Difficulty: Easy)

Per serving: Kcal 208, Fat: 16g, Net Carbs: 4g, Protein: 11g

Ingredients

- 3/4 cup shredded Mozzarella cheese
- 1 Big Egg
- 2 tbsp of Almond Flour
- 2 tbsp of besti erythritol
- 1/2 tbsp melted butter
- 1/2 tsp of cinnamon
- 1 tbsp melted butter
- 1/2 tsp of vanilla extract
- 3/4 tsp of cinnamon
- 1/4 cup of besti erythritol

Instructions

Preheat waffle iron for around 5 minutes. Microwave cream cheese for around 30 seconds. Add the rest of the ingredients except the toppings. Pour mixture that covers the surface of the waffle maker. Cook for around 4 minutes. Take out and place on a plate and repeat with the rest of the batter. To prepare churro chaffles, mix cinnamon and erythritol for topping. Brush chaffles using butter after they are cooked and sprinkle with topping.

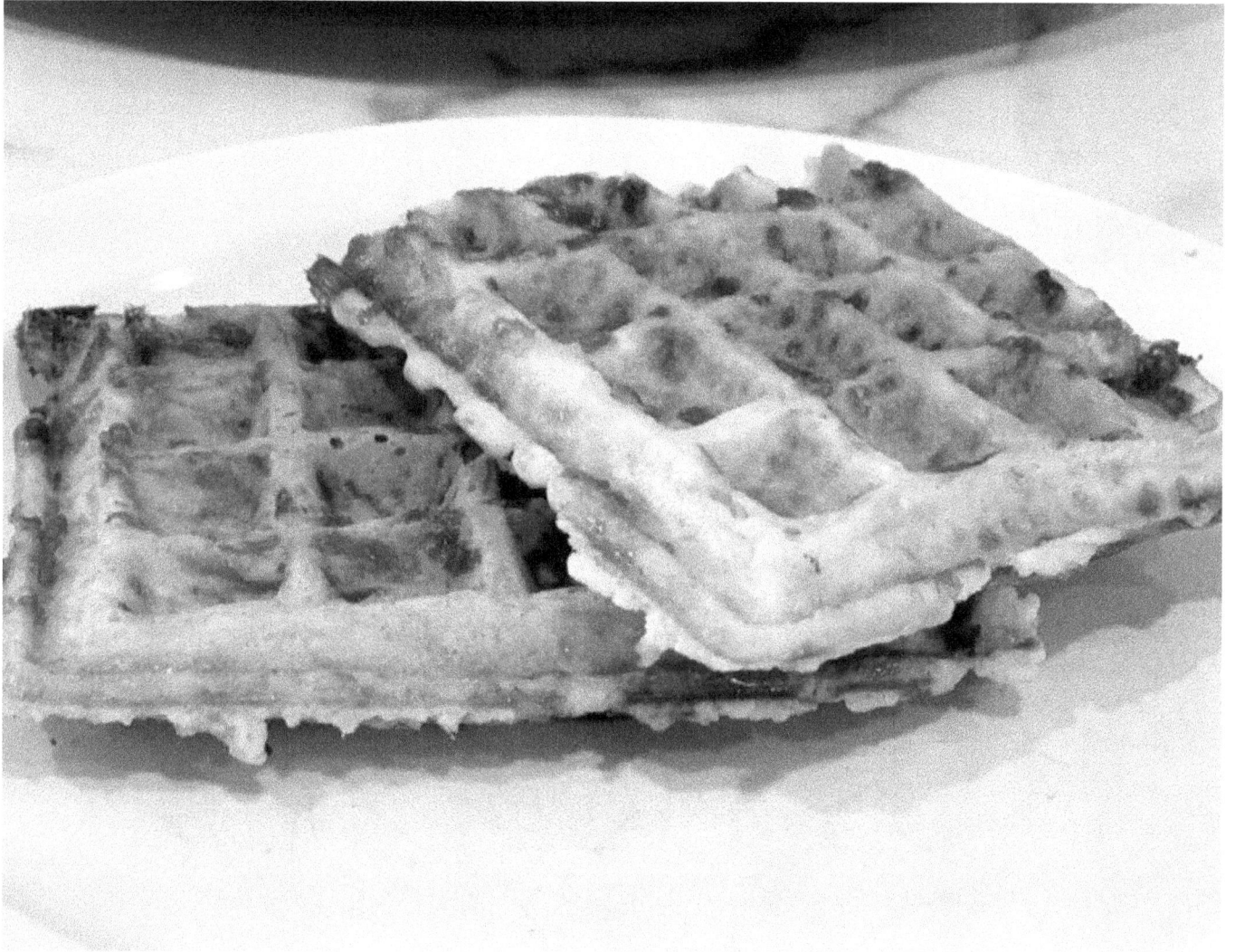

8 CHEESE CHAFFLES

(Ready in about 8 minutes | Serving 2 | Difficulty: Easy)

Per serving: Kcal 208, Fat: 16g, Net Carbs: 4g, Protein: 11g

Ingredients

- 1 Egg
- 1/2 oz of Cream cheese
- 1/2 cup shredded Mozzarella cheese
- 2 1/2 tbsp of Besti Erythritol
- 2 tbsp of pumpkin puree
- 1/2 tbsp of Pumpkin pie spice
- 3 tsp of Coconut Flour

Instructions

Preheat waffle iron for around 5 minutes. Microwave cream cheese for around 30 seconds. Add the rest of the ingredients except the toppings. Pour mixture that covers the surface of the waffle maker. Cook for around 4 minutes. Take out and place on a plate and repeat with the rest of the batter.

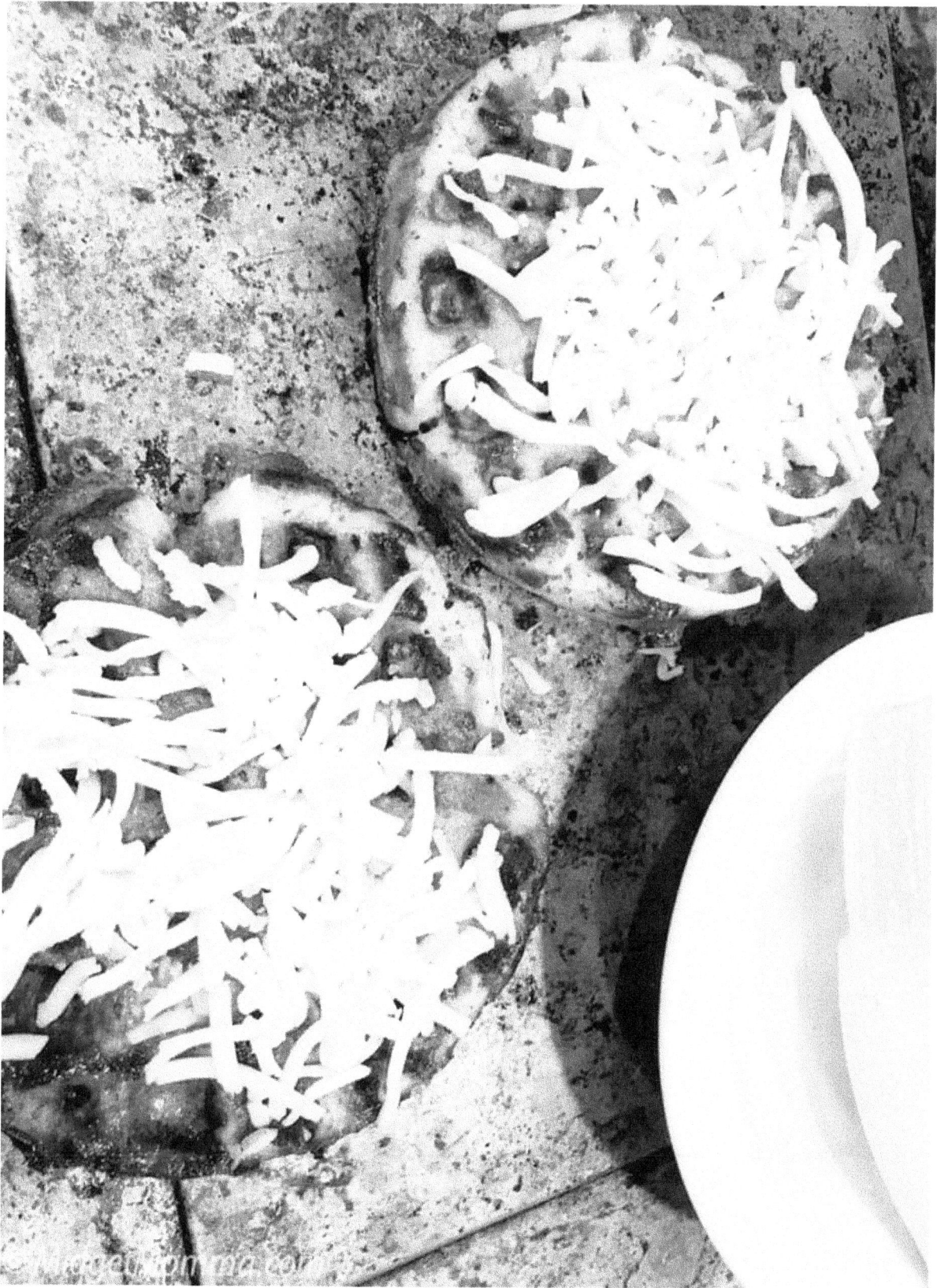

9 SPICY CHAFFLES

(Ready in about 8 minutes | Serving 2 | Difficulty: Easy)

Per serving: Kcal 208, Fat: 16g, Net Carbs: 4g, Protein: 11g

Ingredients

- 1 Egg
- 1 oz of Cream cheese
- 1 cup shredded Cheddar cheese
- 1/2 tbsp of Jalapenos
- 2 tbsp of Bacon bits

Instructions

Preheat waffle iron for around 5 minutes. Microwave cream cheese for around 30 seconds. Add the rest of the ingredients except the toppings. Pour mixture that covers the surface of the waffle maker. Cook for around 4 minutes. Take out and place on a plate and repeat with the rest of the batter.

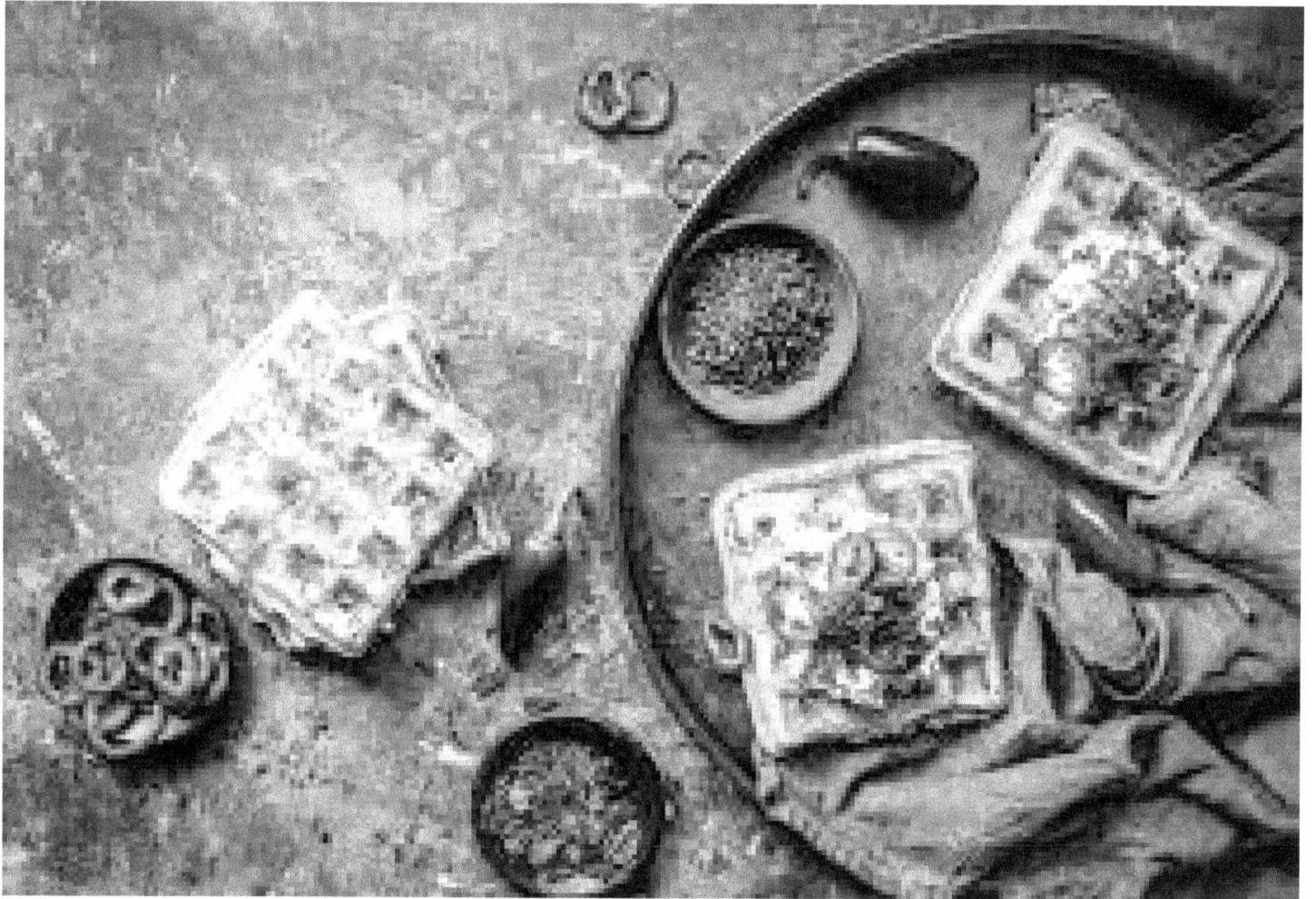

10 DOUBLE CHOCOLATE CHAFFLES

(Ready in about 5 minutes | Serving 1 | Difficulty: Easy)

Per serving: Kcal 197, Fat: 23.3g, Net Carbs: 11.3g, Protein: 24.3g

Ingredients

- 1 egg
- 1 tbsp of granulated sweetener
- 1/2 cup grated mozzarella
- 1 tsp of vanilla
- 1 tbsp of chocolate chips
- 2 tbsp of almond meal/flour
- 1 tsp of heavy cream
- 2 tbsp unsweetened cocoa powder

Instructions

Add all the ingredients to a bowl and mix. Preheat the waffle maker. Spray with oil and pour half amount of batter into the maker. Cook for around 4 minutes. Sprinkle with toppings and enjoy.

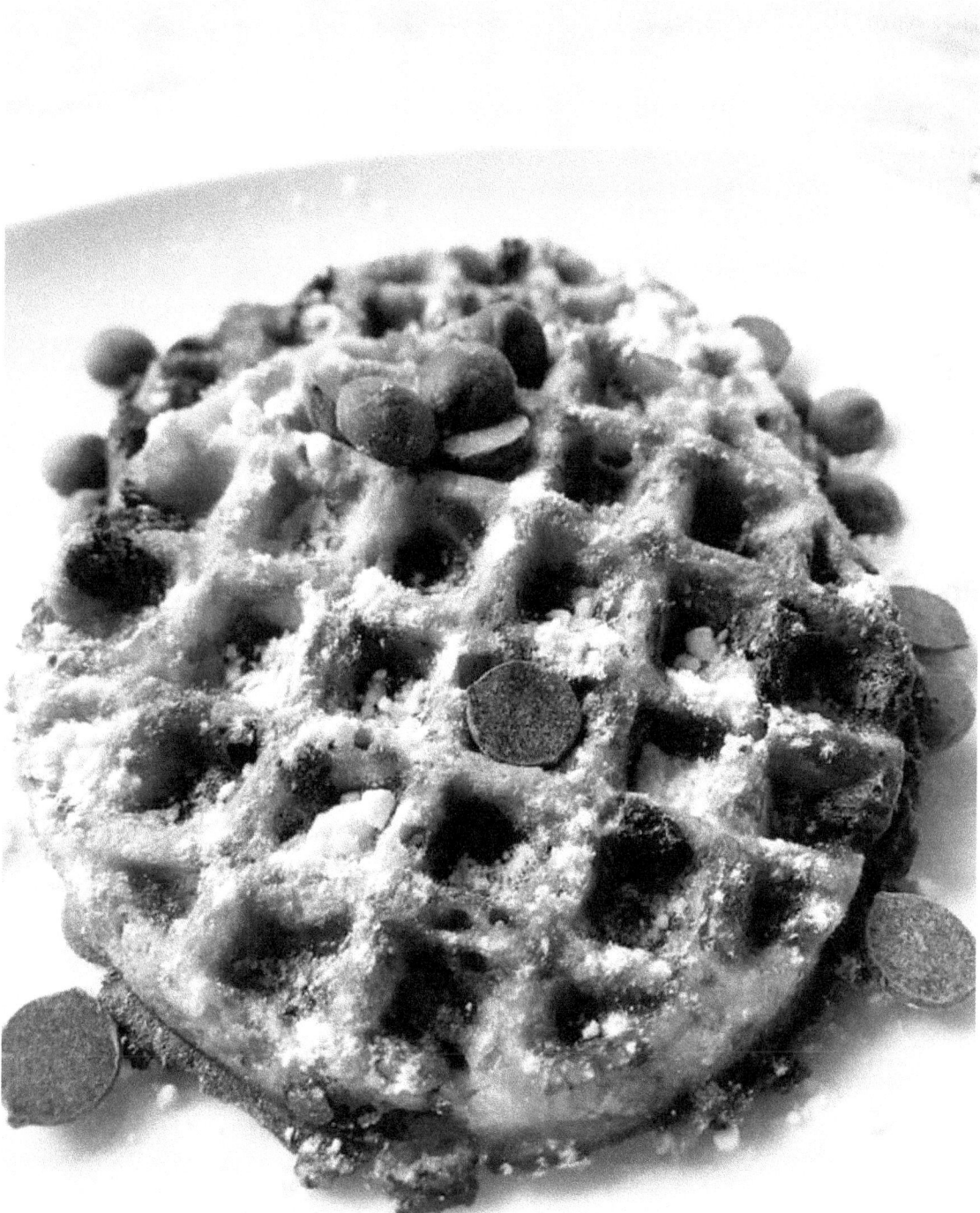

137

11 VANILLA CHAFFLES

(Ready in about 10 minutes | Serving 1 | Difficulty: Easy)

Per serving: Kcal 184, Fat: 20.1g, Net Carbs: 5.4g, Protein: 22.2g

Ingredients

- 1/2 cup of grated mozzarella
- 1 tbsp of granulated sweetener
- 1 eggs
- 1 tsp of vanilla extract
- 1 tbsp of chocolate chips
- 2 tbsp of almond flour

Instructions

Combine all the ingredients in a bowl. Preheat the waffle maker and spray it using oil once it is hot. Pour half amount of batter in the maker and cook for around 4 minutes. Remove and do the same with the rest of the batter. Top and enjoy.

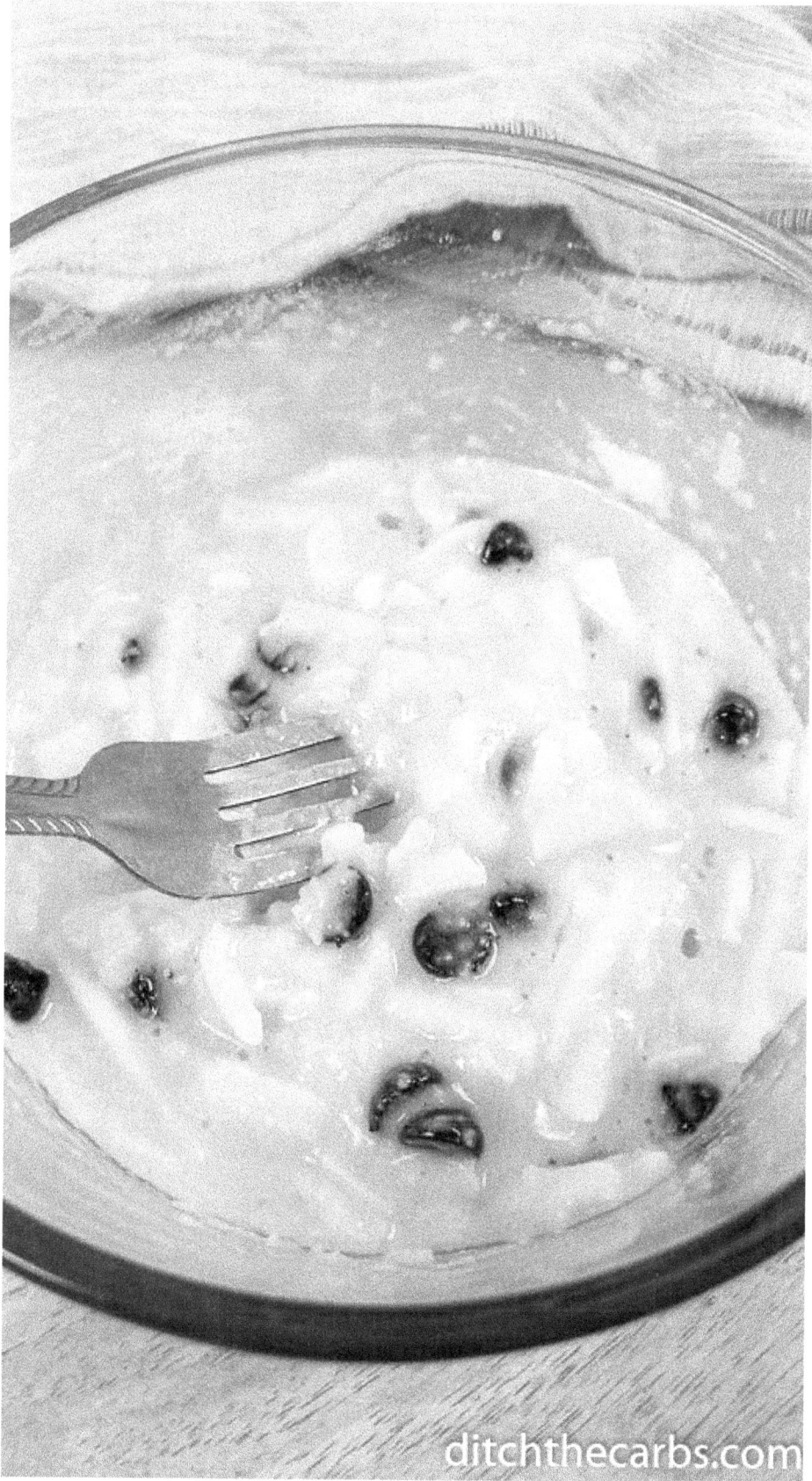

12 LEMON CURD CHAFFLE

(Ready in about 50 minutes | Serving 3 | Difficulty: Hard)

Per serving: Kcal 302, Fat: 24g, Net Carbs: 6g, Protein: 15g

Ingredients

- 3 eggs
- one batch of lemon curd
- 4 ounces softened cream cheese
- 1 tsp of vanilla extract
- 1 tbsp sweetener low carb
- 3/4 cup shredded mozzarella cheese
- 1 tsp of baking powder
- 3 tbsp of coconut flour
- 1/3 tsp of salt

Instructions

Prepare lemon curd according to package instructions. Heat the maker and spray oil. Mix baking powder, salt and coconut flour in a bowl. Add the rest of the ingredients to another bowl and beat using a hand blender. Mix the two bowls mixture and pour in the maker. Cook for around 5 minutes. Top using lemon curd.

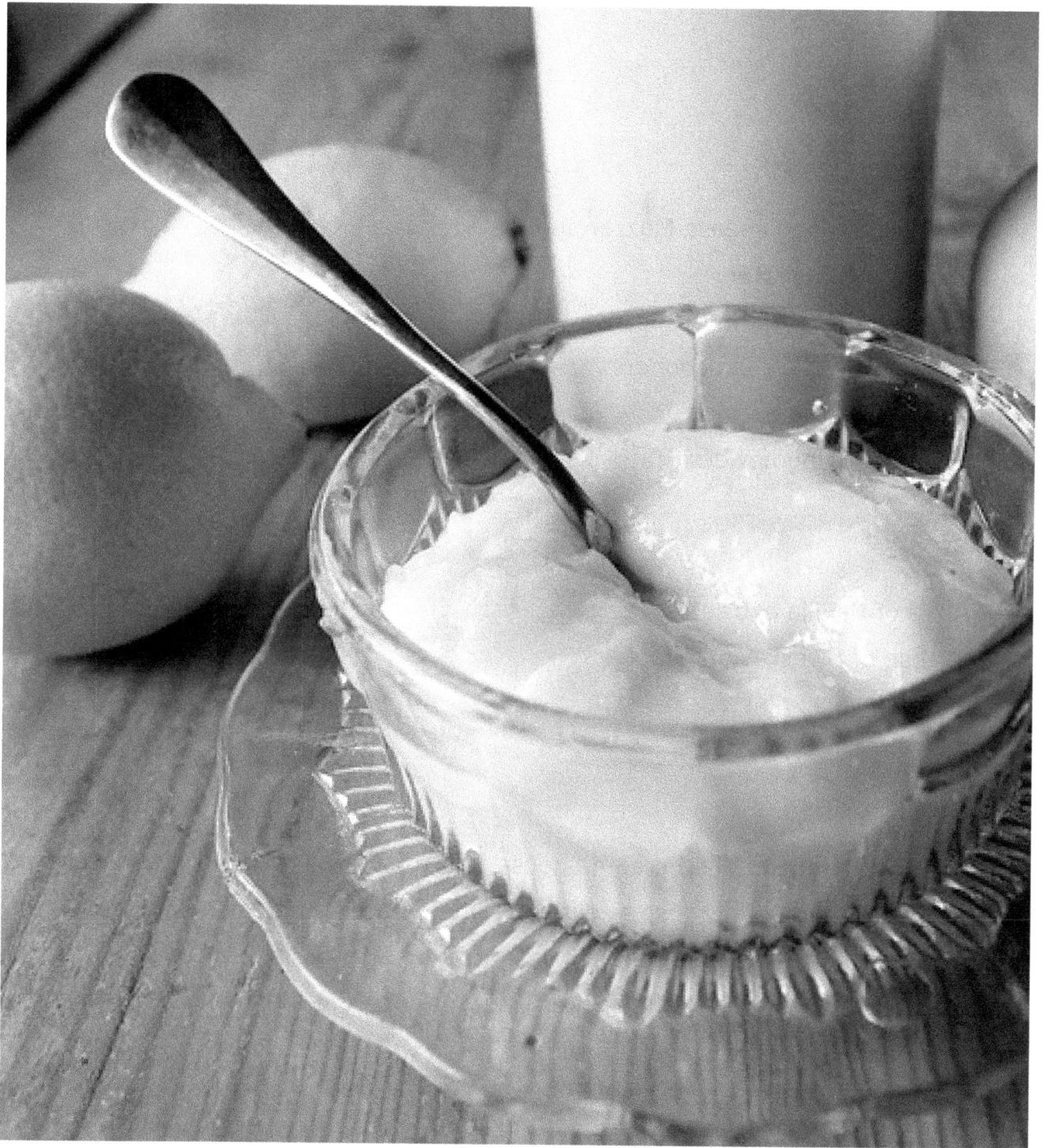

13 GLAZED DONUT

(Ready in about 15 minutes | Serving 3 | Difficulty: Easy)

Per serving: Kcal 246, Fat: 17g, Net Carbs: 2g, Protein: 14g

Ingredients

For chaffles

- 1/2 cup shredded cheese Mozzarella
- 2 tbsp of whey protein
- 1 ounce of Cream Cheese
- 2 tbsp of Swerve confectioners
- 1/2tsp of Vanilla extract
- 1/2tsp of Baking powder
- 1 Egg

For glaze

- 1/2tsp of Vanilla extract
- 3-4 tbsp of Swerve confectioners
- 2 tbsp of whipping cream

Instructions

Preheat the waffle maker. Add cream cheese and mozzarella in a bowl and microwave for around 30 seconds. Add 2 tbsp sweetener, whey protein and baking powder and mix. Add dough to a bowl and break an egg into it and add vanilla. Stir to form a smooth mixture. Add batter to the waffle maker and cook for around 5 minutes. Beat glaze ingredients in a bowl and top chaffles with it.

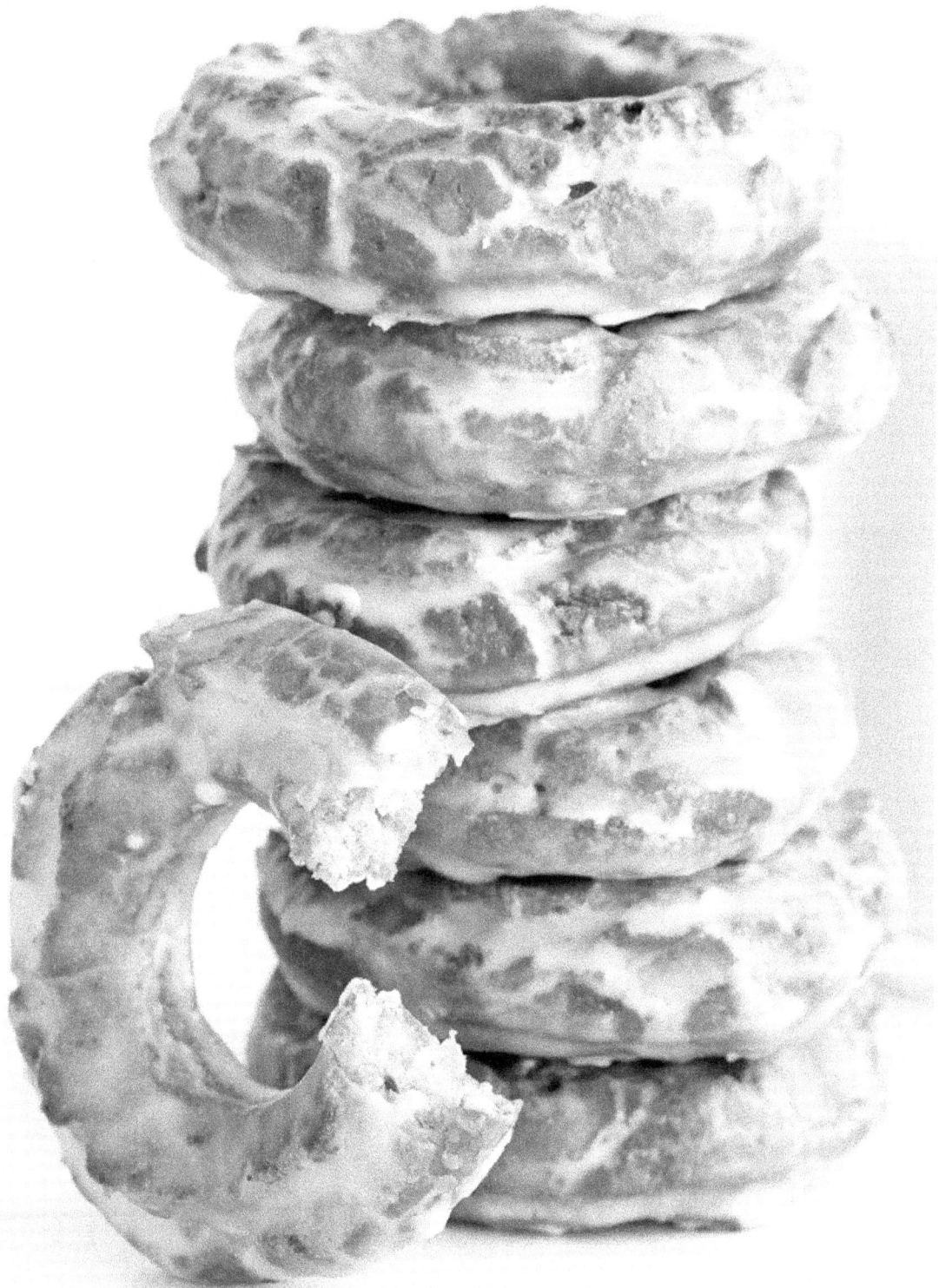

14 NUT-FREE CHAFFLES

(Ready in about 30 minutes | Serving 3 | Difficulty: Easy)

Per serving: Kcal 195, Fat: 15.1g, Net Carbs: 31.5g, Protein: 8.5g

Ingredients

Batter

- 1/2 cup shredded cheese mozzarella
- 1/4 tsp of vanilla extract
- 2 tbsp of SunButter
- 2 tbsp of fruit sweetener
- 1 egg
- 2 tsp of cinnamon
- 1 tbsp of coconut flour
- ⅛ tsp of baking powder

Frosting

- 1 tbsp of cream cheese
- 1/4 cup of fruit sweetener
- 3/4 tbsp of butter, melted
- 1 tbsp of coconut milk unsweetened
- 1/4 tsp of vanilla extract

Coating

- 1 tsp of fruit sweetener
- 1 tsp of cinnamon

Instructions

Preheat the waffle iron. Mix batter ingredients in a bowl and place aside. Mix frosting ingredients except for coconut milk in a bowl and whisk until smooth. Add coconut milk and mix again. Place aside. Coat iron with cooking spray and add batter. Cook for around 4 minutes. Sprinkle with sweetener and cinnamon.

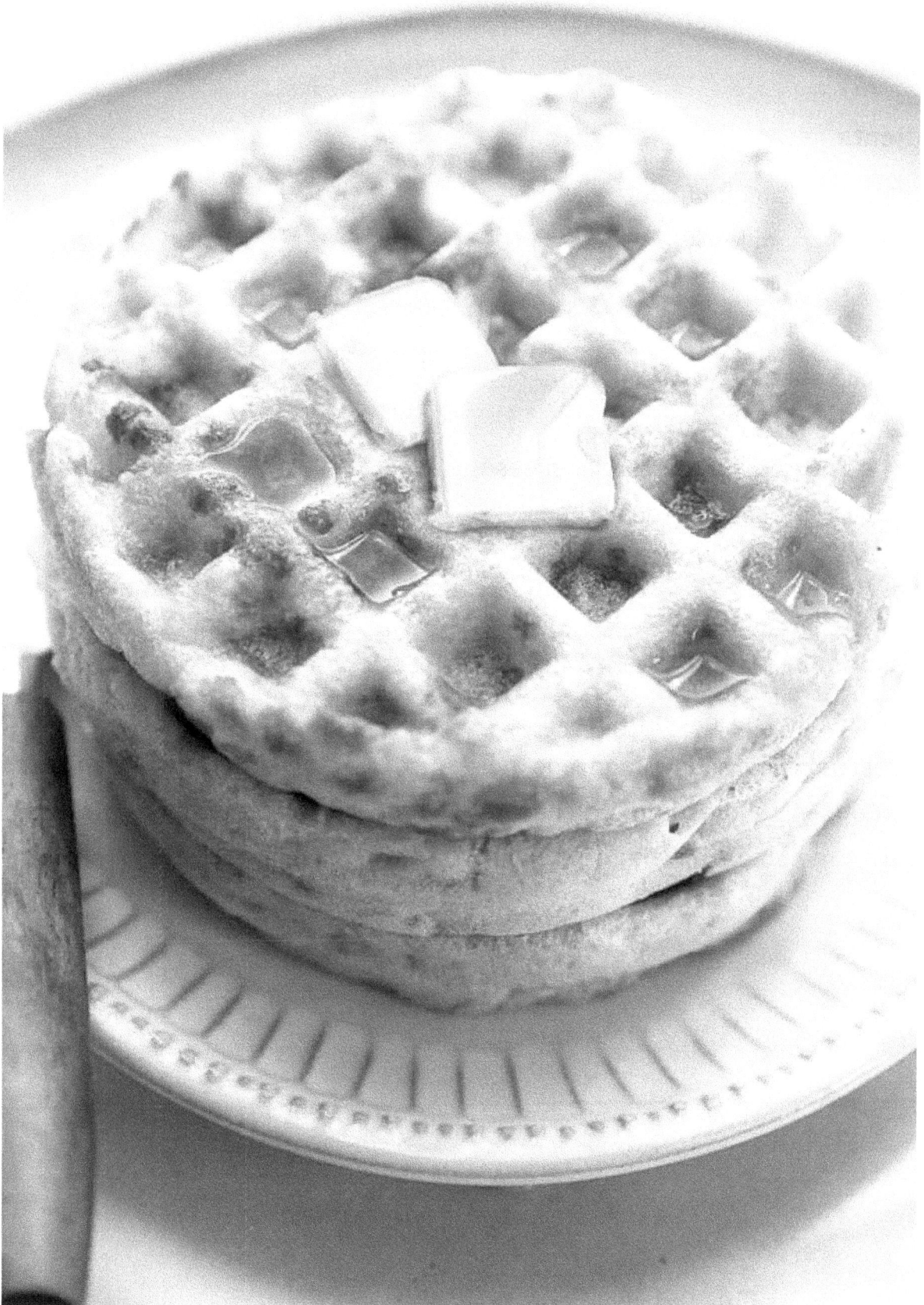

15 CHICKEN CHAFFLE

(Ready in about 19 minutes | Serving 2 | Difficulty: Easy)

Per serving: Kcal 675, Fat: 52g, Net Carbs: 8g, Protein: 44g

Ingredients

- 1/4 cup of almond flour
- 1/4 cup crumbled feta cheese
- 2 eggs
- 1 tsp of baking powder
- 1/2 cup shredded chicken
- 1/4 cup of Hot Sauce
- 1/4 cup shredded mozzarella cheese
- 3/4 cup shredded cheddar cheese
- 1/4 cup diced celery

Instructions

Mix almond flour and baking powder in a bowl. Preheat iron and spray using cooking spray. Beat eggs in a bowl and add hot sauce. Combine thoroughly and pour flour mixture. Combine and add grated cheeses. Fold in chicken. Pour in the maker and cook for around 4 minutes. Top with celery and feta.

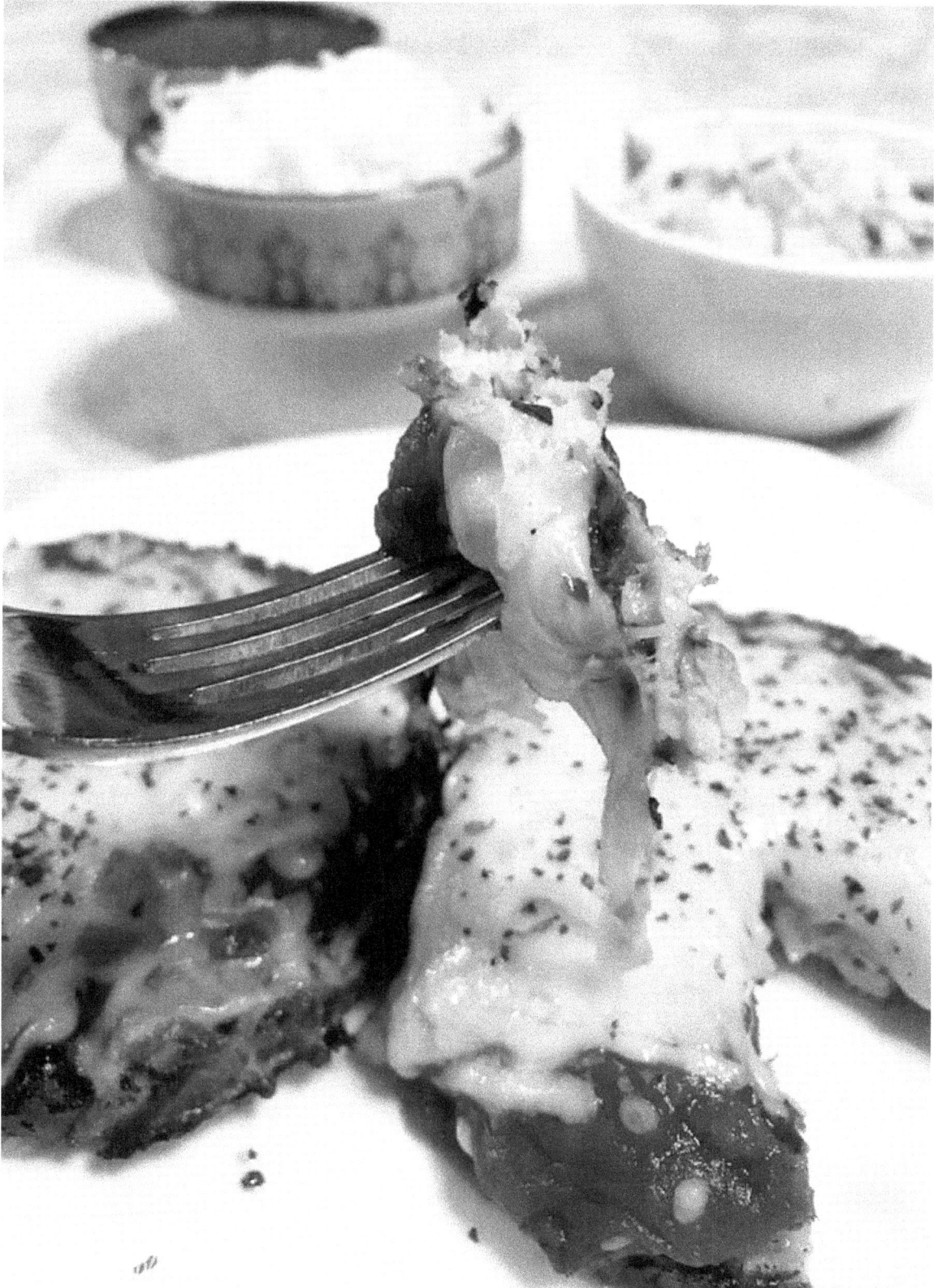

16 CHAFFLE SANDWICH

(Ready in about 13 minutes | Serving 1 | Difficulty: Easy)

Per serving: Kcal 238, Fat: 18g, Net Carbs: 2g, Protein: 17g

Ingredients

For chaffles

- 1/2 cup shredded Cheddar cheese
- 1 egg

For sandwich

- 1 tbsp of mayonnaise
- 2 slices of tomato
- 2 strips of bacon
- 3 pieces of lettuce

Instructions

Preheat the maker and mix cheese and egg in a bowl. Pour batter into the maker and cook for around 4 minutes. Do it in 2 batches. Cook bacon in pan paced on the moderate flame until it gets crispy. Drain using paper towels and form a sandwich using tomato, mayonnaise and lettuce.

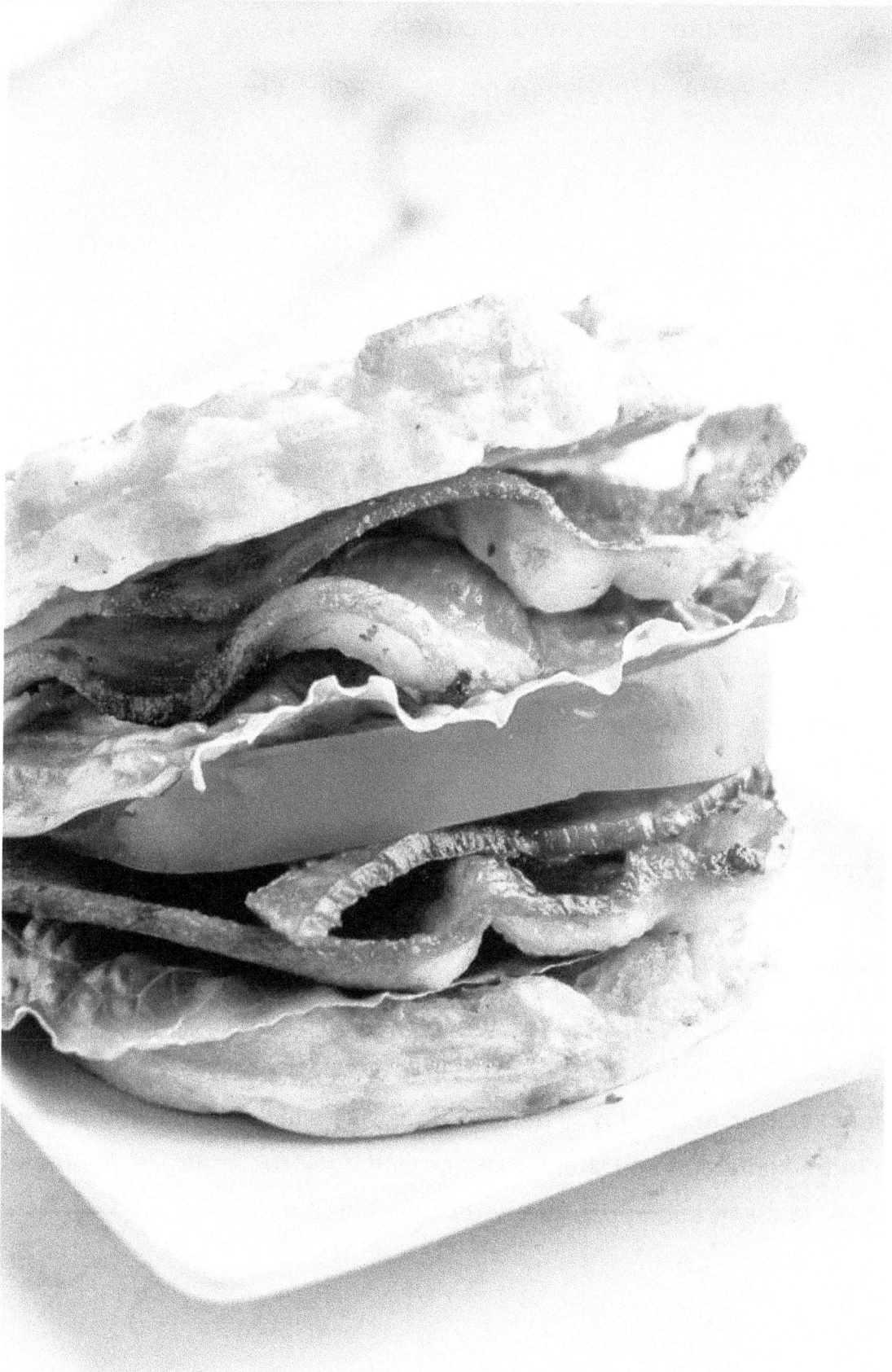

17 SAUSAGE GRAVY CHAFFLE

(Ready in about 15 minutes | Serving 2 | Difficulty: Easy)

Per serving: Kcal 212, Fat: 17g, Net Carbs: 3g, Protein: 11g

Ingredients

For Chaffle

- 1/2 cup grated mozzarella cheese
- 1 egg
- 1 tsp of coconut flour
- 1/4 tsp of baking powder
- 1 tsp of water
- Salt

For Gravy

- 3 tbsp of chicken broth
- 1/4 cup browned breakfast sausage
- 2 tbsp of whipping cream
- dash of garlic powder
- 2 tsp softened cream cheese
- pepper

Instructions

Preheat the maker and coat using cooking spray. Add all ingredients to a bowl and mix. Pour half amount to mixture into the maker and cook for around 4 minutes. Repeat with the remaining batter and enjoy. Prepare breakfast sausage and add in the pan with remaining ingredients and boil. Reduce flame and cook for around 7 minutes to thicken it. Add pepper and salt and spoon gravy on top of chaffles.

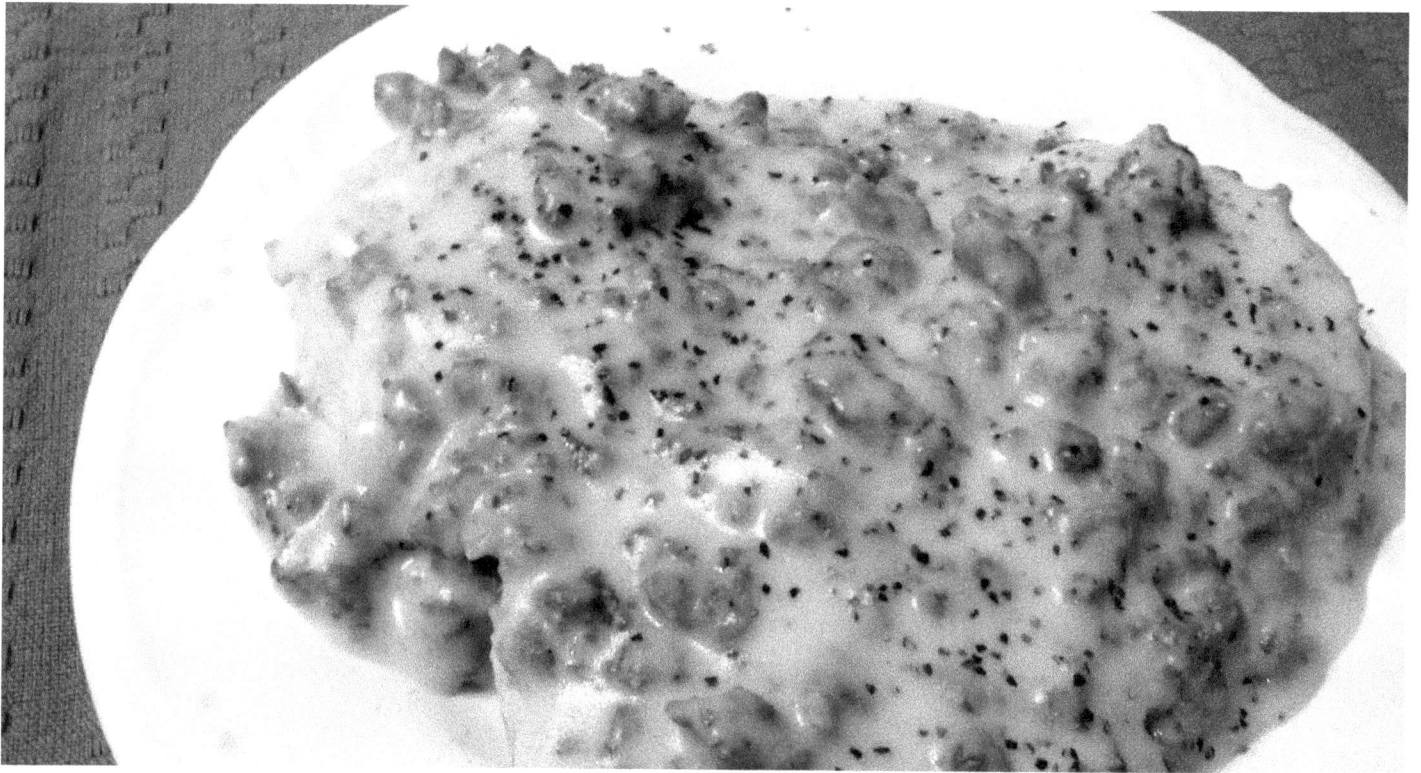

18 EGGS BENEDICT

(Ready in about 30 minutes | Serving 2 | Difficulty: Easy)

Per serving: Kcal 844, Fat: 78g, Net Carbs: 5g, Protein: 32g

Ingredients

For Chaffles

- 1/2 cup of mozzarella cheese
- 2 tbsp of almond flour
- 2 whites of eggs
- 1 tbsp of sour cream

For Hollandaise

- 2 tbsp of lemon juice
- 4 yolks of eggs
- 1/2 cup of salted butter

For Eggs

- 1 tbsp of white vinegar
- 3 ounces of deli ham
- 2 eggs

Instructions

Whisk eggs in a bowl and with the rest of the ingredients and blend. Preheat the waffle maker. Spray using cooking spray and add half the mixture. Cook for around 7 minutes. Make hollandaise sauce by forming a double broiler. Boil water and warm butter in the microwave. Add egg to bowl of the boiler. Boil and add hot butter while the pot is carried to a boil. Cook until egg thickens and take out of the bowl. Drizzle lemon juice and place aside. Warm chaffle using toaster and top with ham slices, 2 tbsp hollandaise sauce and one egg.

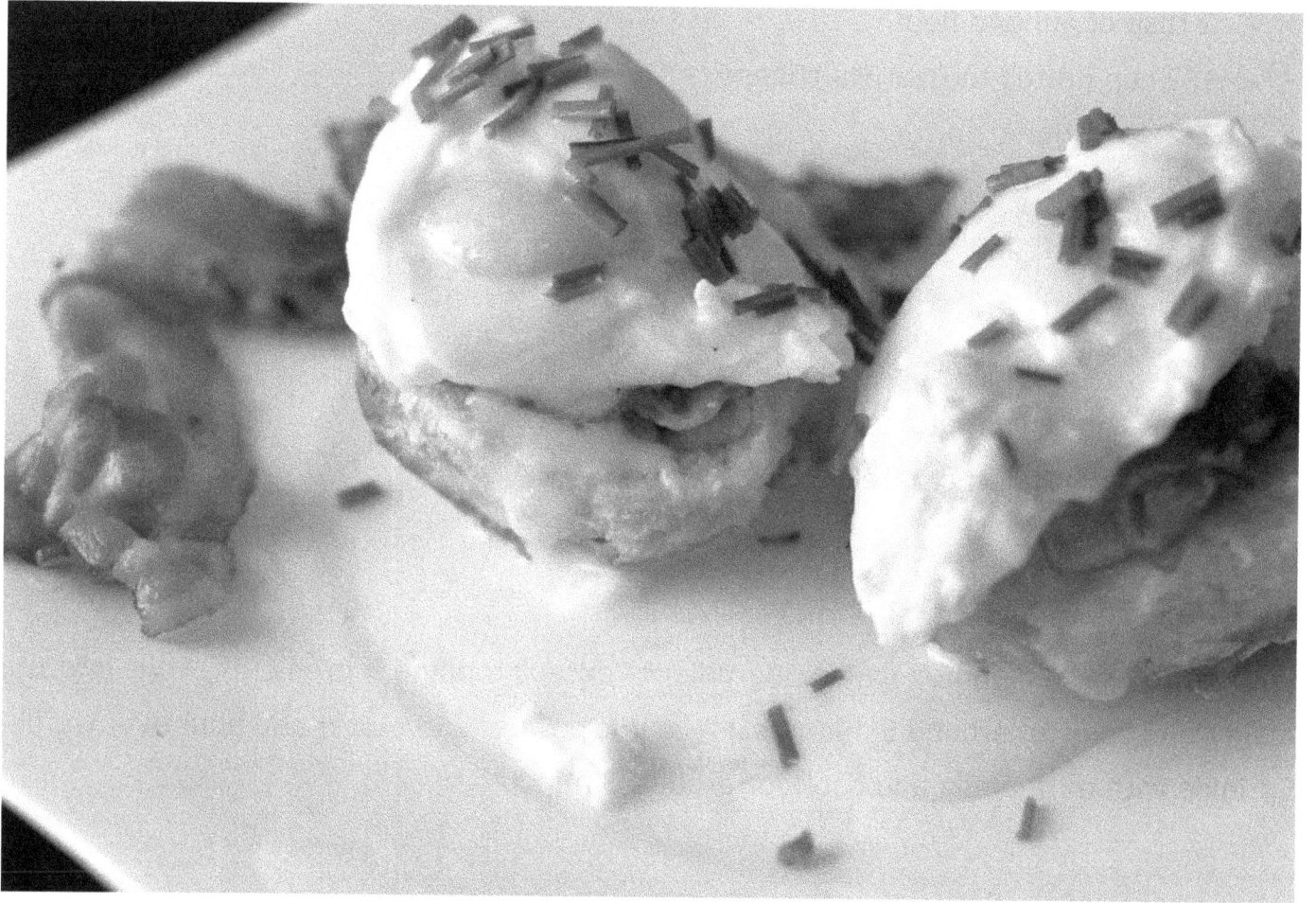

19 GARLIC CHAFFLE

(Ready in about 10 minutes | Serving 8 | Difficulty: Easy)

Per serving: Kcal 74, Fat: 6.5g, Net Carbs: 0.9g, Protein: 3.4g

Ingredients

- 1 egg
- 2 tbsp of almond flour
- 1/2 cup grated mozzarella cheese
- 1/2tsp of garlic powder
- 1/2tsp of salt
- 1/2tsp of oregano

Topping

- 1/2tsp of garlic powder
- 2 tbsp softened butter
- 1/4 cup grated mozzarella cheese

Instructions

Preheat the maker and oil it. Mix ingredients except topping ingredients. Pour into the maker and cook for around 5 minutes. Mix garlic powder and butter and pour over waffle. Sprinkle with mozzarella and cook for around 3 minutes.

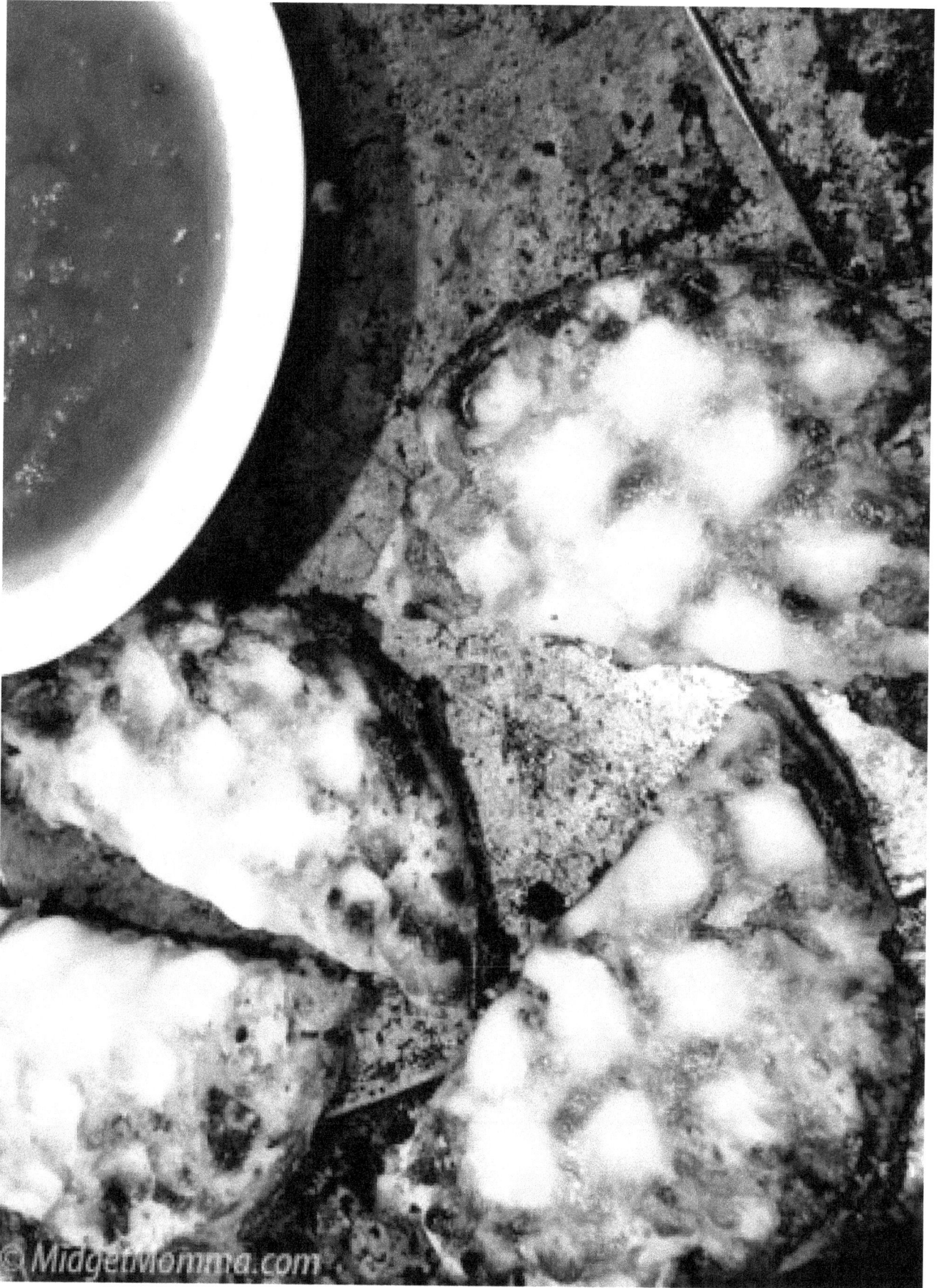

© MidgetMomma.com

20 TACO CHAFFLE

(Ready in about 13 minutes | Serving 1 | Difficulty: Easy)

Per serving: Kcal 258, Fat: 19g, Net Carbs: 4g, Protein: 18g

Ingredients

- 1/4 cup shredded jack cheese
- 1 white of egg
- 1/4 cup shredded cheddar cheese
- 1 tsp of coconut flour
- 3/4 tsp of water
- 1/4 tsp of baking powder
- pinch of salt
- 1/8 tsp of chili powder

Instructions

Preheat the maker and oil it. Combine everything in a bowl and spoon half amount of mixture in the maker. Cook for around 4 minutes. Remove the chaffle shell and place it aside. Repeat with the remaining batter. Turn the pan and position shells of the chaffle among cups to make a shell of taco.

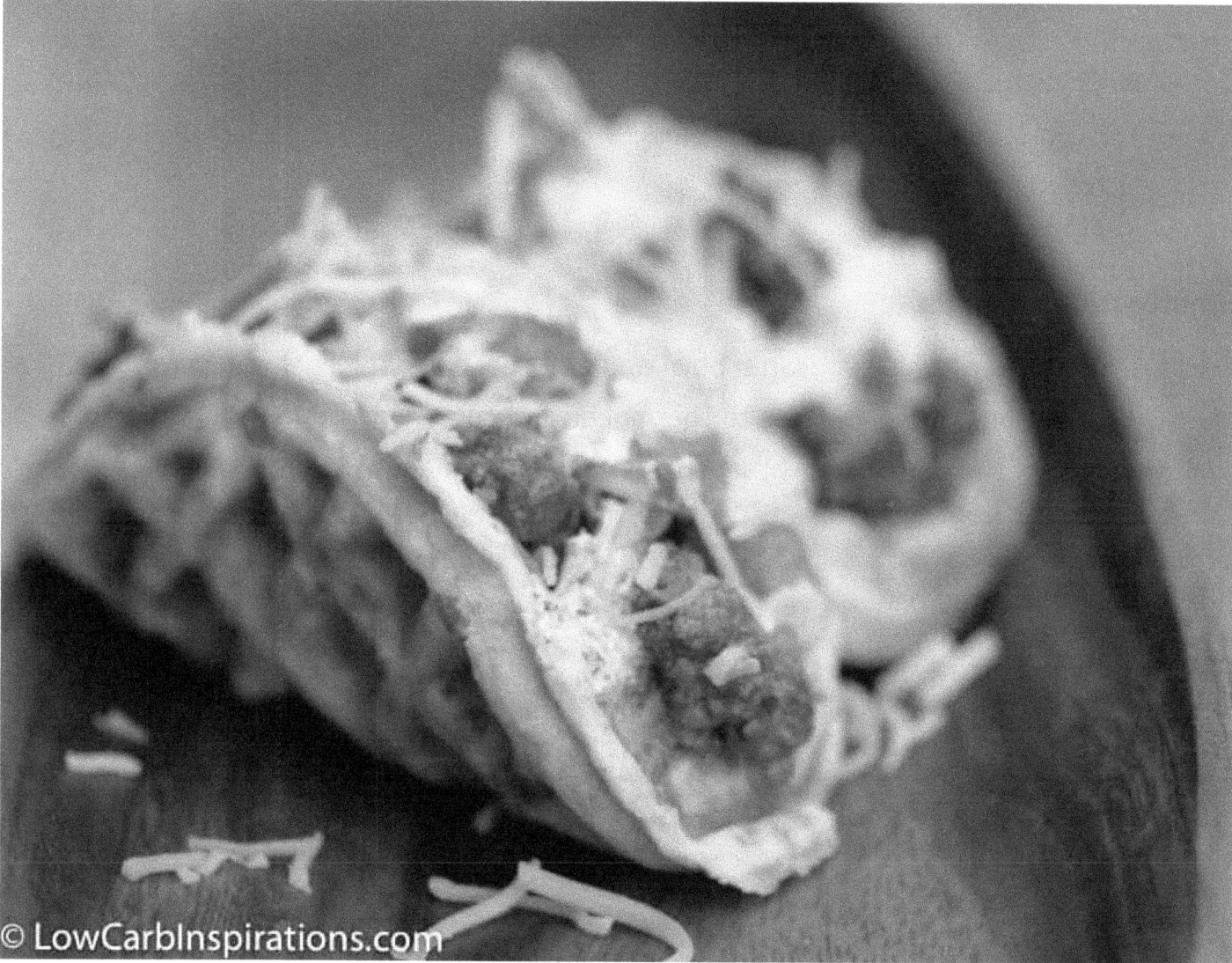

© LowCarbInspirations.com

21 PIZZA CHAFFLE

(Ready in about 8 minutes | Serving 2 | Difficulty: Easy)

Per serving: Kcal 76, Fat: 4.3g, Net Carbs: 4.1g, Protein: 5.5g

Ingredients

- 1 egg
- Pinch of Italian seasoning
- 1/2 cup shredded mozzarella cheese
- 1 tbsp of pizza sauce

Instructions

Preheat the maker. Whisk eggs in a bowl and add seasonings. Mix shredded cheese in a bowl. Add half amount of mixture to the maker and cook for around 4 minutes. Repeat with the rest of the batter and with 1 tbsp pizza sauce and pepperoni.

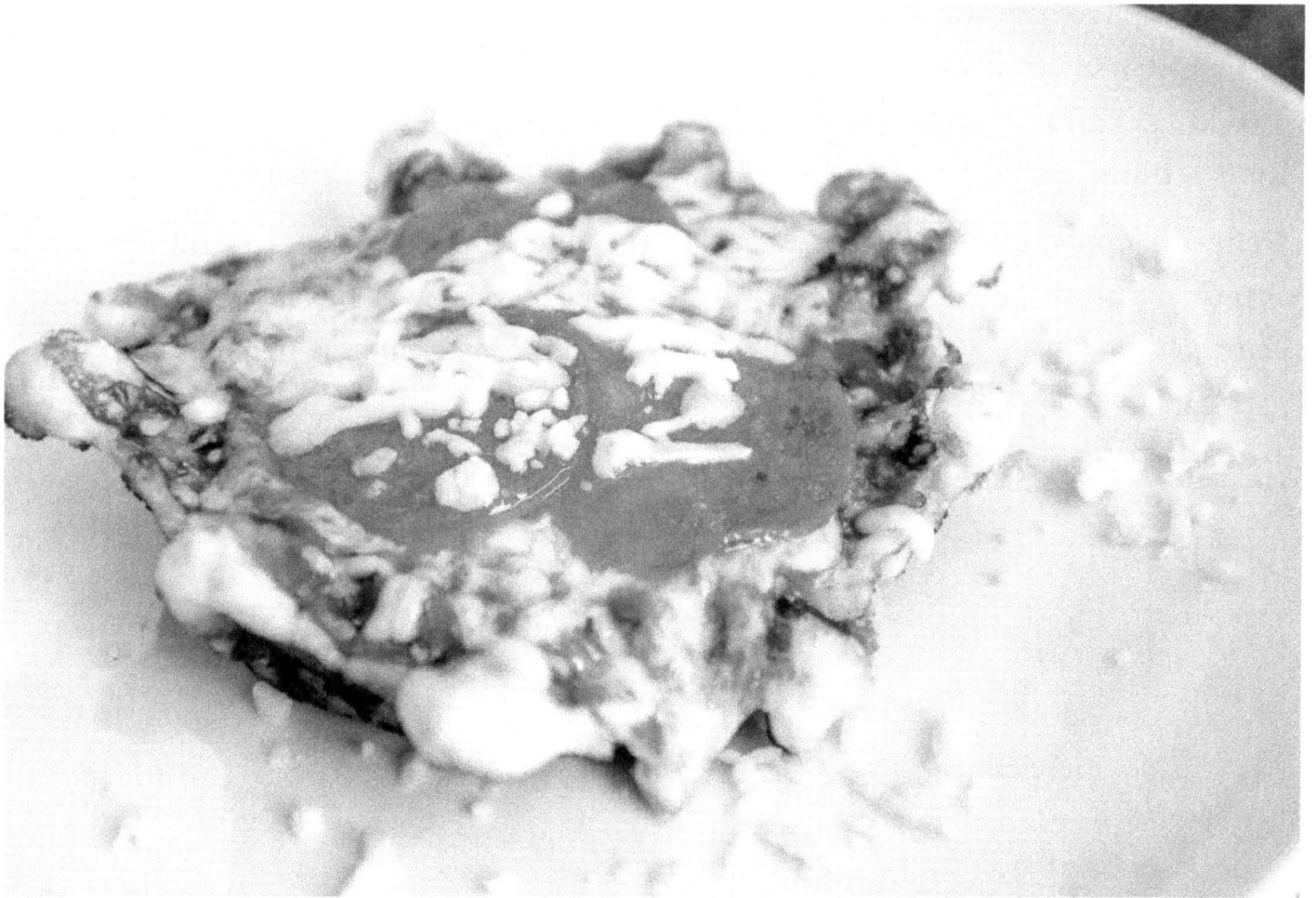

22 PARMESAN CHAFFLES

(Ready in about 6 minutes | Serving 1 | Difficulty: Easy)

Per serving: Kcal 352, Fat: 24g, Net Carbs: 2g, Protein: 14g

Ingredients

- 1 beaten egg
- 1/2 cup of mozzarella cheese shredded
- 1/4 cup of Parmesan cheese grated
- 1/4tsp of garlic powder
- 1 tsp of Italian seasoning

Instructions

Preheat the waffle maker. Add all the ingredients except mozzarella and parmesan cheese in a bowl and mix. Mix the cheese in a bowl and spray waffle sung cooking spray. Pour half amount of mixture in the maker and cook for around 5 minutes. Top using parmesan and enjoy.

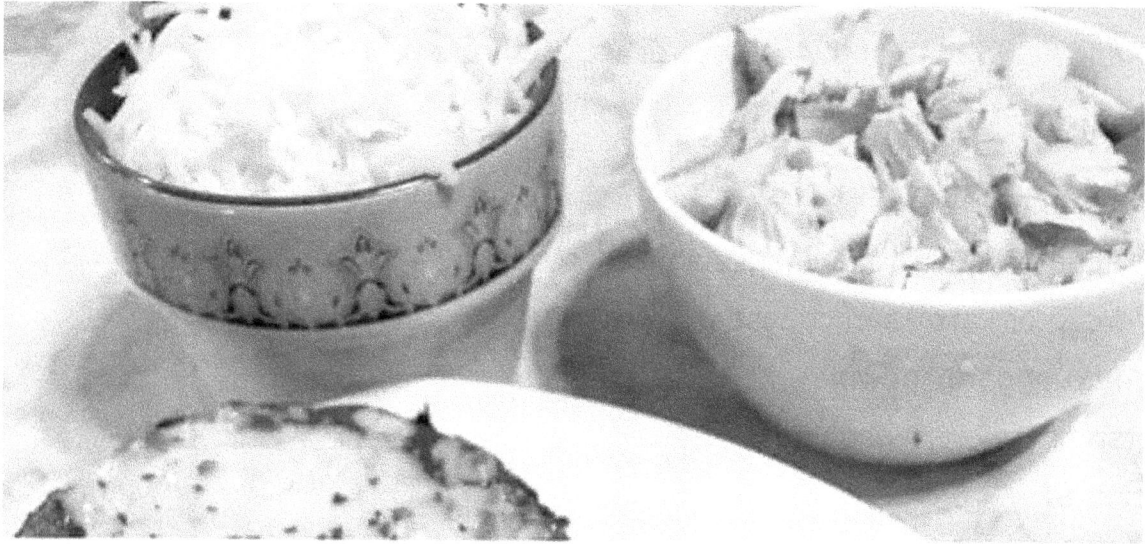

CHICKEN PARMESAN Chaffle

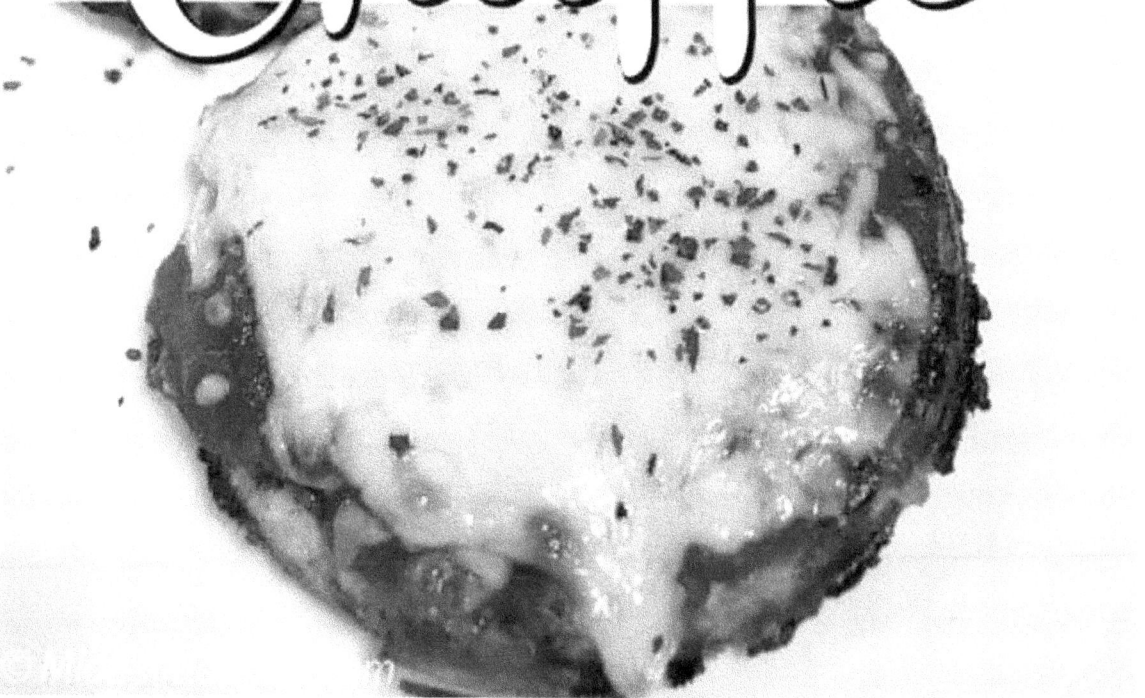

23 ITALIAN CHAFFLE

(Ready in about 6 minutes | Serving 1 | Difficulty: Easy)

Per serving: Kcal 352, Fat: 24g, Net Carbs: 2g, Protein: 14g

Ingredients

- 1 beaten egg
- 1/2 cup of mozzarella cheese shredded
- 1/4 cup of Parmesan cheese grated
- 1/4tsp of garlic powder
- 1 tsp of Italian seasoning

Instructions

Preheat the waffle maker. Add all the ingredients except mozzarella and parmesan cheese in a bowl and mix. Mix the cheese in a bowl and spray waffle sung cooking spray. Pour half amount of mixture in the maker and cook for around 5 minutes. Top using parmesan and add lettuce, cold cuts, tomato.

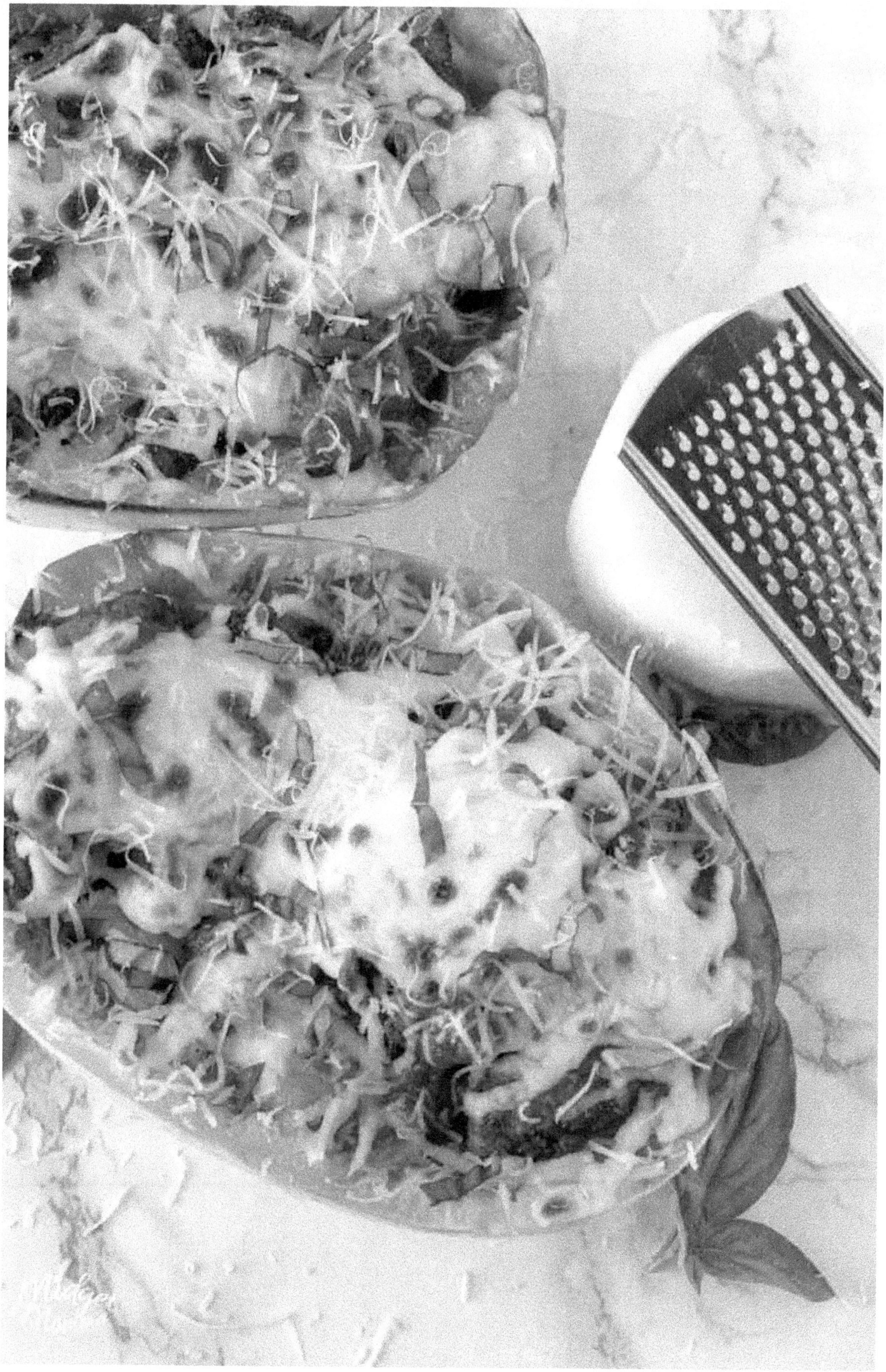

24 CHAFFLE BREADSTICKS

(Ready in about 6 minutes | Serving 1 | Difficulty: Easy)

Per serving: Kcal 352, Fat: 24g, Net Carbs: 2g, Protein: 14g

Ingredients

- 1 beaten egg
- 1/2 cup of mozzarella cheese shredded
- Marinara sauce
- 1/4 cup of Parmesan cheese grated
- 1/4tsp of garlic powder
- 1 tsp of Italian seasoning

Instructions

Preheat the waffle maker. Add all the ingredients except mozzarella and parmesan cheese in a bowl and mix. Mix the cheese in a bowl and spray waffle sung cooking spray. Pour half amount of mixture in the maker and cook for around 5 minutes. Top using parmesan and dice into 4 sticks and enjoy with Marinara Sauce.

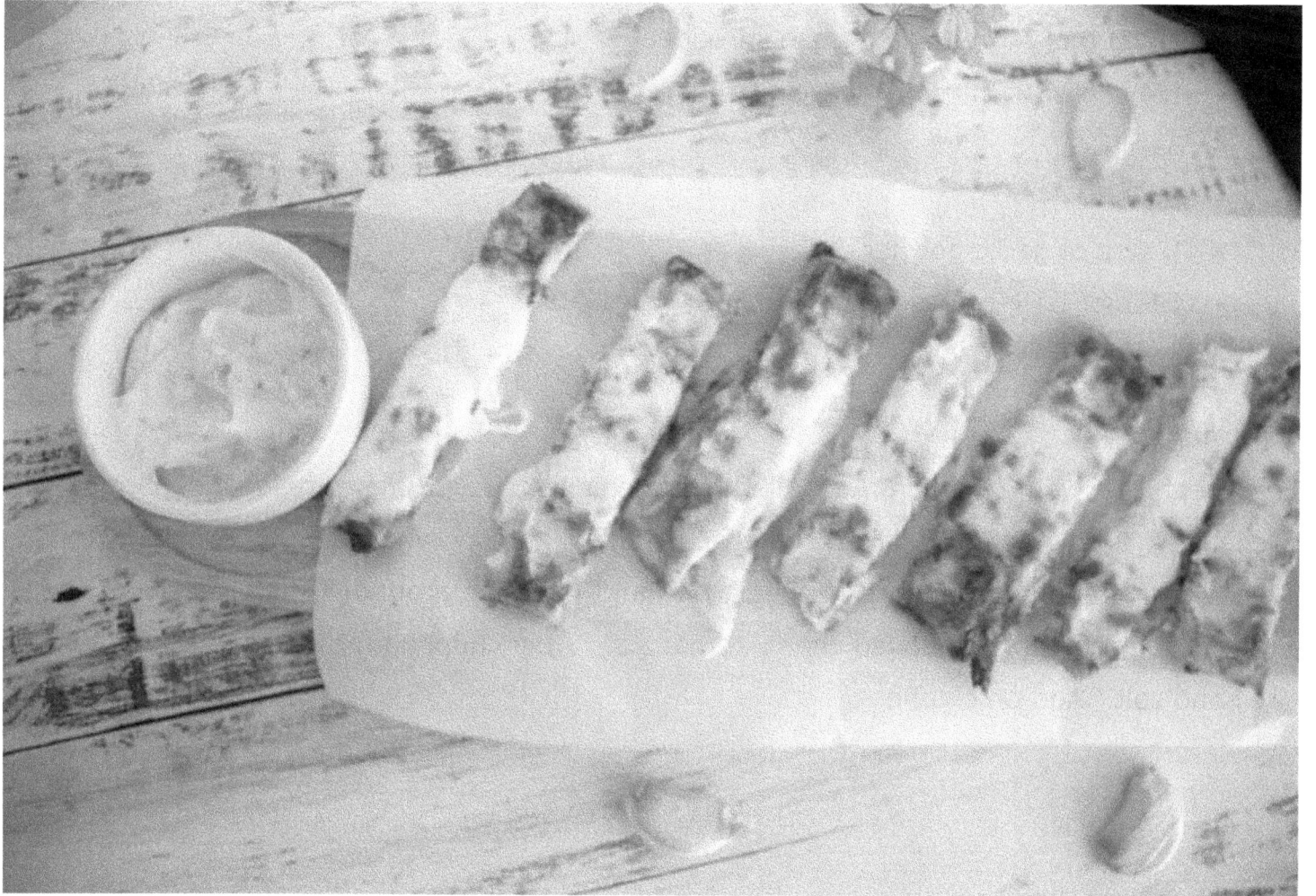

25 CHAFFLE BRUSCHETTA

(Ready in about 6 minutes | Serving 1 | Difficulty: Easy)

Per serving: Kcal 352, Fat: 24g, Net Carbs: 2g, Protein: 14g

Ingredients

- 1 beaten egg
- 1/2 cup of mozzarella cheese shredded
- 1/4 cup of Parmesan cheese grated
- Basil
- Olive oil
- 1/4tsp of garlic powder
- 1 tsp of Italian seasoning

Instructions

Preheat the waffle maker. Add all the ingredients except mozzarella and parmesan cheese in a bowl and mix. Mix the cheese in a bowl and spray waffle sung cooking spray. Pour half amount of mixture in the maker and cook for around 5 minutes. Top using parmesan and mix 4 chopped cherry tomatoes, ½ tsp chopped fresh basil, drop of olive oil and salt. Add on chaffle.

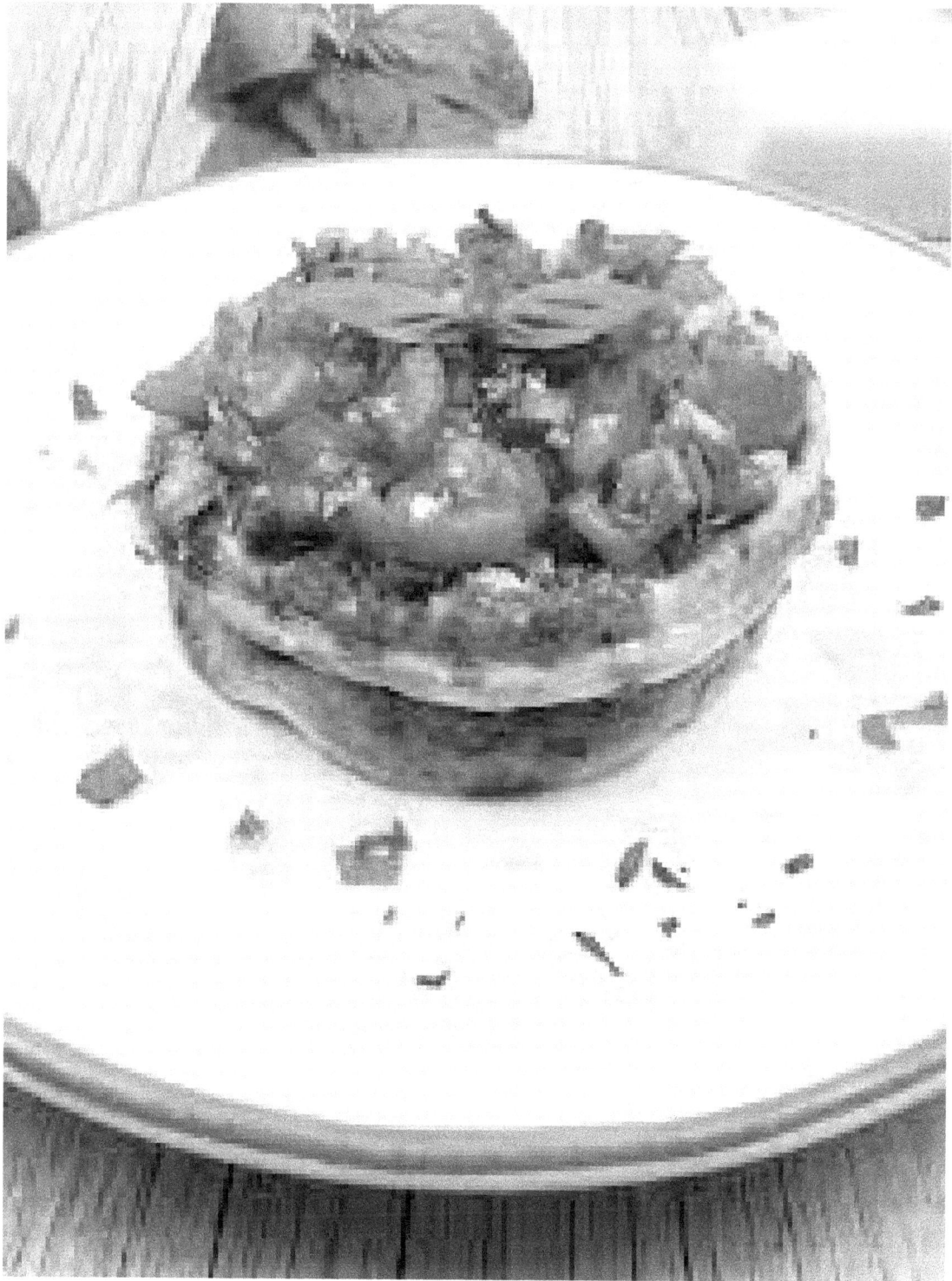

26 CAULIFLOWER CHAFFLES

(Ready in about 9 minutes | Serving 2 | Difficulty: Easy)

Per serving: Kcal 246, Fat: 16g, Net Carbs: 7g, Protein: 20g

Ingredients

- 1/4 tsp of Garlic Powder
- 1 cup of riced cauliflower
- 1/4 tsp of Ground Black Pepper
- 1/4 tsp of Kosher Salt
- 1/2 tsp of Italian seasoning
- 1 Eggs
- 1/2 cup of mozzarella cheese shredded
- 1/2 cup of parmesan cheese shredded

Instructions

Blend all ingredients except the cauliflower mixture and parmesan cheese in a blender and sprinkle half parmesan in the maker. Pour mixture in maker and top with cauliflower mixture and rest of parmesan. Cook for around 5 minutes.

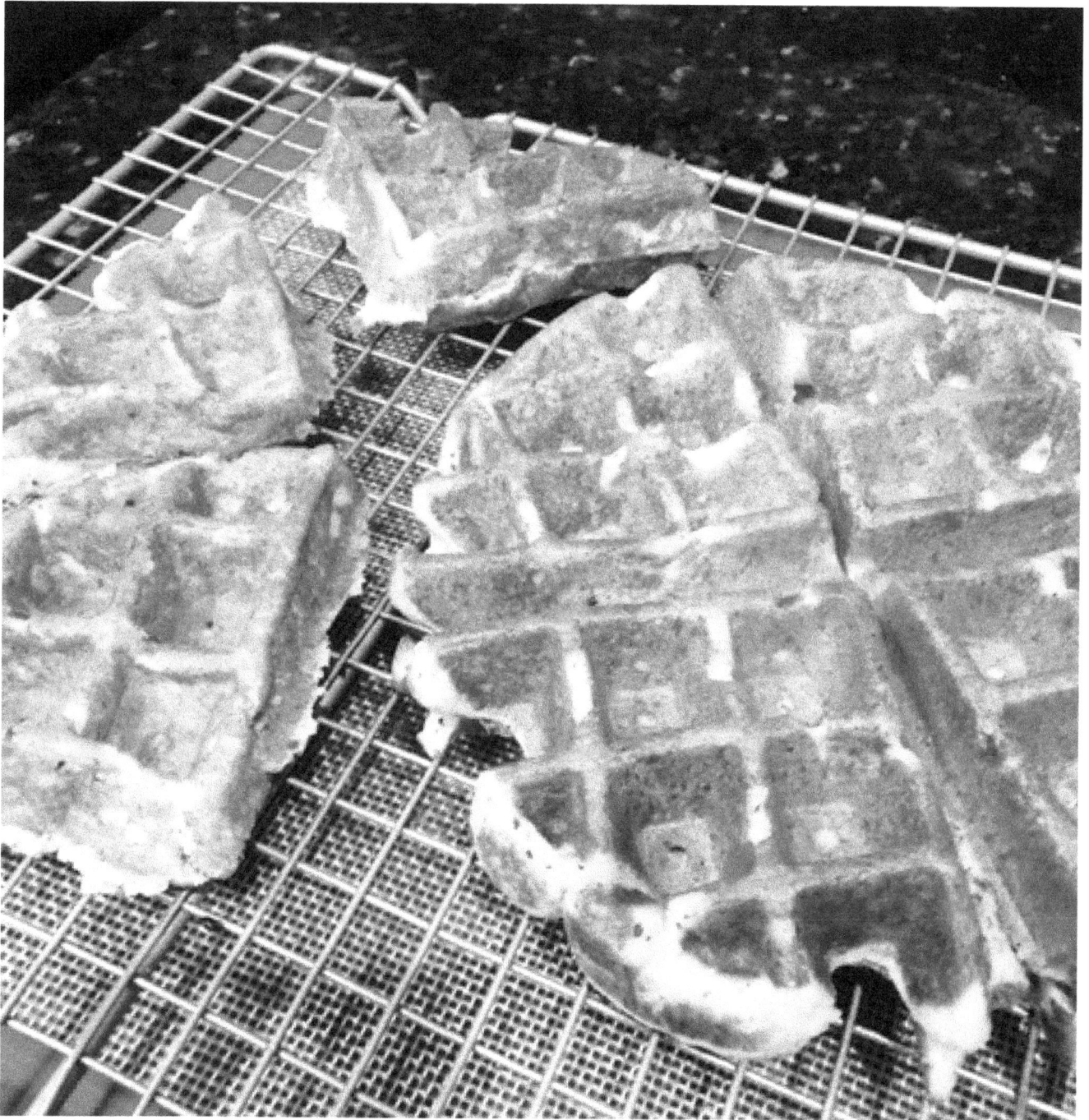

27 ZUCCHINI CHAFFLES

(Ready in about 15 minutes | Serving 2 | Difficulty: Easy)

Per serving: Kcal 194, Fat: 13g, Net Carbs: 4g, Protein: 16g

Ingredients

- 1 beaten Egg
- 1/2 tsp Black Pepper Ground
- 1 cup grated Zucchini
- 1/2 cup of parmesan cheese shredded
- 1 tsp chopped Dried Basil
- 1/4 cup of mozzarella cheese shredded
- 3/4 tsp divided Kosher Salt

Instructions

Sprinkle 1/4 tsp salt on zucchini. Beat egg in a bowl and add mozzarella, zucchini, 1/2 tsp salt, basil and pepper. Sprinkle 2 tbsp parmesan on iron and spread a quarter of zucchini mixture on the maker. Top using 2 tbsp parmesan and cook for around 8 minutes. Repeat with the rest of the mixture.

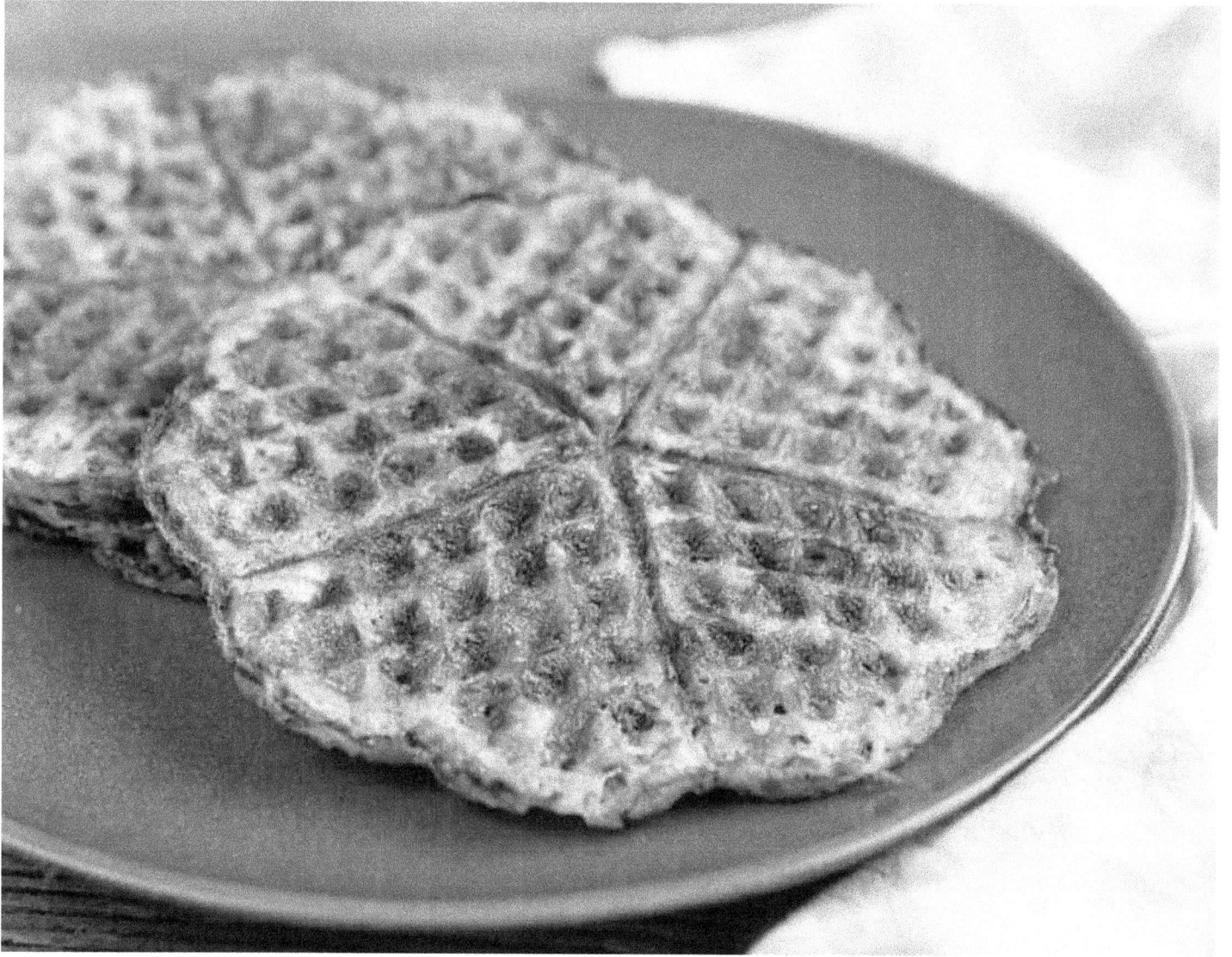

28 PEANUT CHAFFLES

(Ready in about 6 minutes | Serving 2 | Difficulty: Easy)

Per serving: Kcal 264, Fat: 21.6g, Net Carbs: 7.25g, Protein: 9.45g

Ingredients

Chaffle

- 1 Egg
- 1/4 tsp of Baking Powder
- 1 tbsp of Unsweetened Cocoa
- 1 tbsp of Heavy Cream
- 1 tbsp of Powdered Sweetener
- 1/2 tsp of Vanilla Extract
- 1 tsp of Coconut Flour
- 1/2 tsp of Batter Flavor

Butter Filling

- 2 tsp of Powdered Sweetener
- 3 tbsp of Peanut Butter
- 2 tbsp of Heavy Cream

InstructionsPreheat the maker. Combine ingredients of chaffle in a bowl and pour half amount of mixture in maker. Cook for around 5 minutes. Repeat with the rest of the mixture. Blend butter ingredients and spread over chaffles.

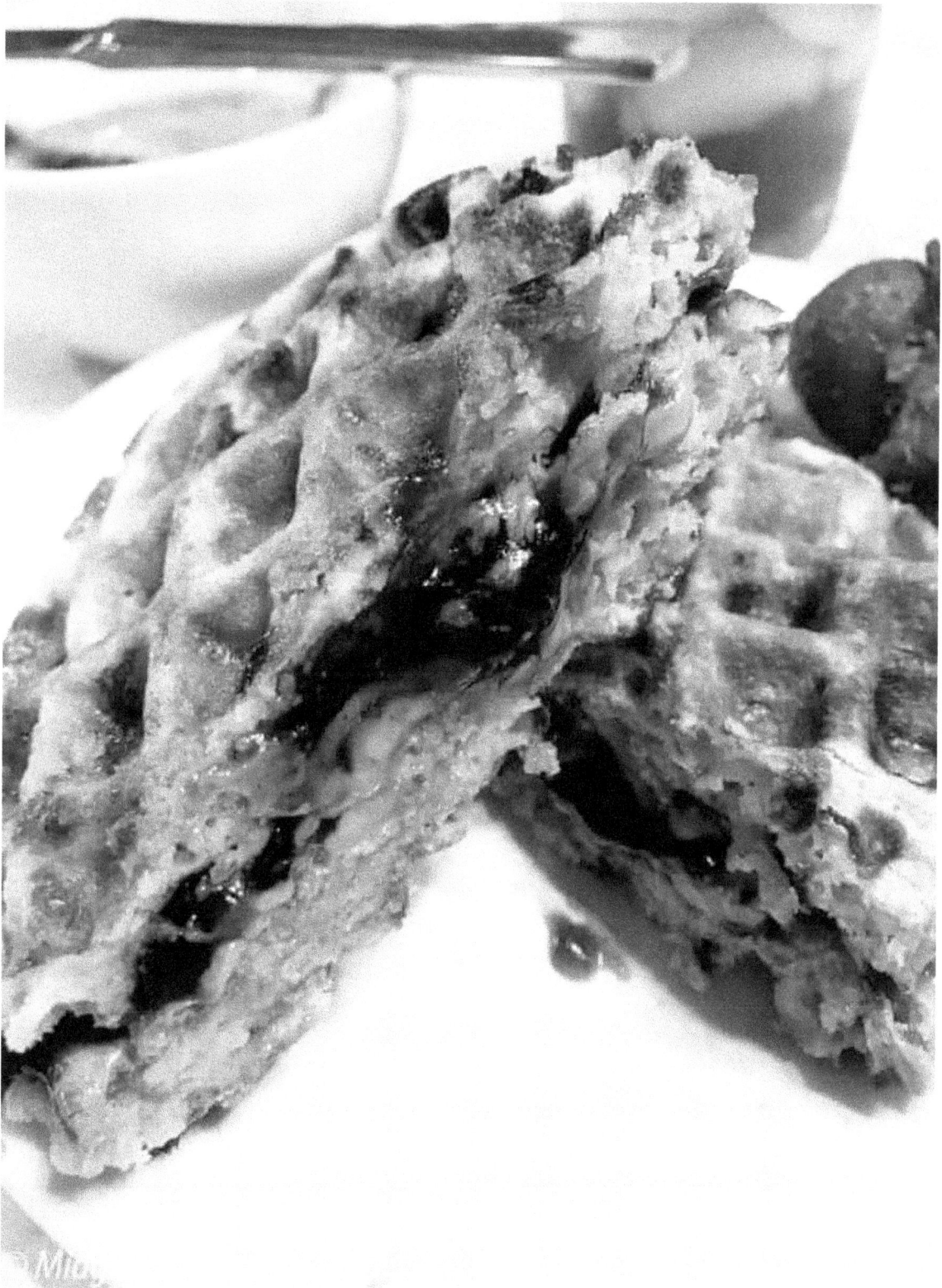

29 EASY CHAFFLE RECIPE

(Ready in about 10 minutes | Serving 2| Difficulty: Easy)

Ingredients

Simple Chaffles

Per serving: Kcal 152, Fat: 8g, Net Carbs: 1g, Protein: 9g

- 1 Egg
- 1/2 Cup of Shredded Cheese Mozarella

Instructions

Add all ingredients to a bowl and whisk to combine. Coat waffle maker using cooking spray and pour half amount of batter into the maker. Cook for around 5 minutes and repeat with the rest of the batter.

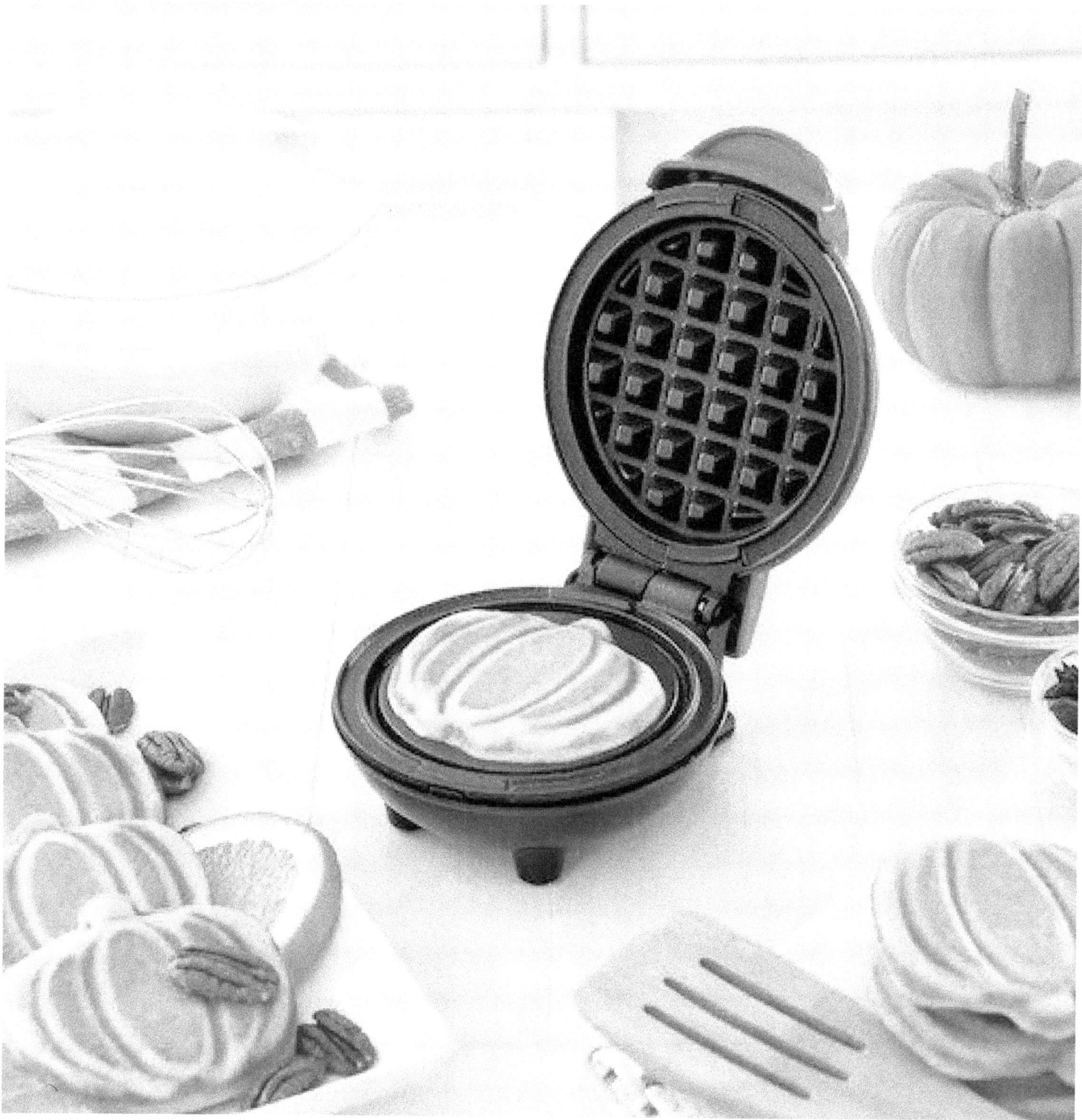

30 SAVORY CHAFFLES

Per serving: Kcal 215, Fat: 16.5g, Net Carbs: 2g, Protein: 12g

- 1 Egg
- 1/2 Cup Shredded Cheese Mozarella
- 1/16 Tsp of Xanthan Gum
- 1/4 Cup of Almond Flour

Instructions

Add all ingredients to a bowl and whisk to combine. Coat waffle maker using cooking spray and pour half amount of batter into the maker. Cook for around 5 minutes and repeat with the rest of the batter.

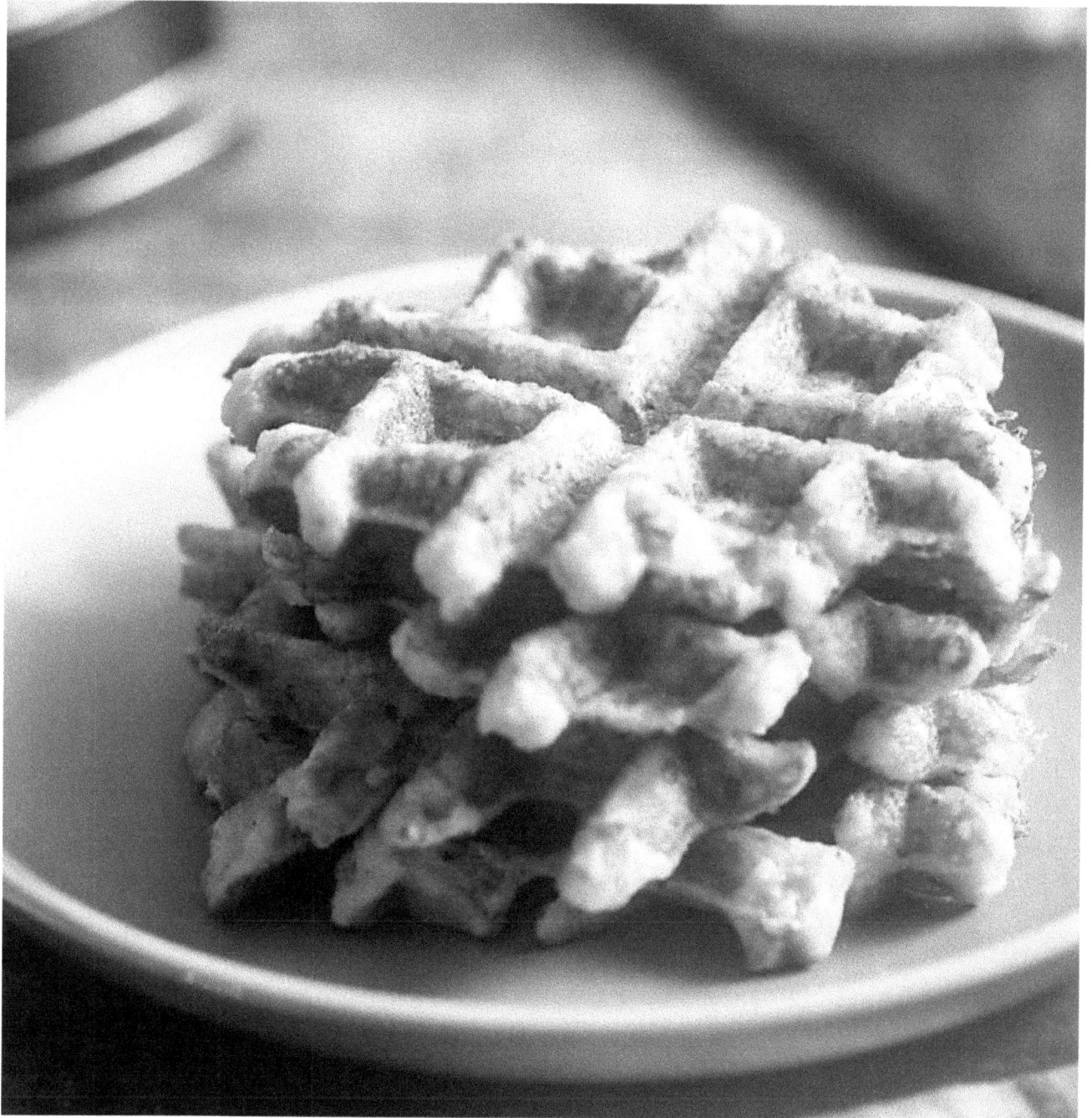

31 SWEET CHAFFLES

Per serving: Kcal 192, Fat: 15gg, Net Carbs: 1.55g, Protein: 15g

- 1 Egg
- 1/2 Cup of Shredded Cheese Mozzarella
- 1/4 Cup of Almond Flour
- 1/16 Tsp of Xanthan Gum
- 2 Tbsp of Confectioners Swerve

Instructions

Add all ingredients to a bowl and whisk to combine. Coat waffle maker using cooking spray and pour half amount of batter into the maker. Cook for around 5 minutes and repeat with the rest of the batter.

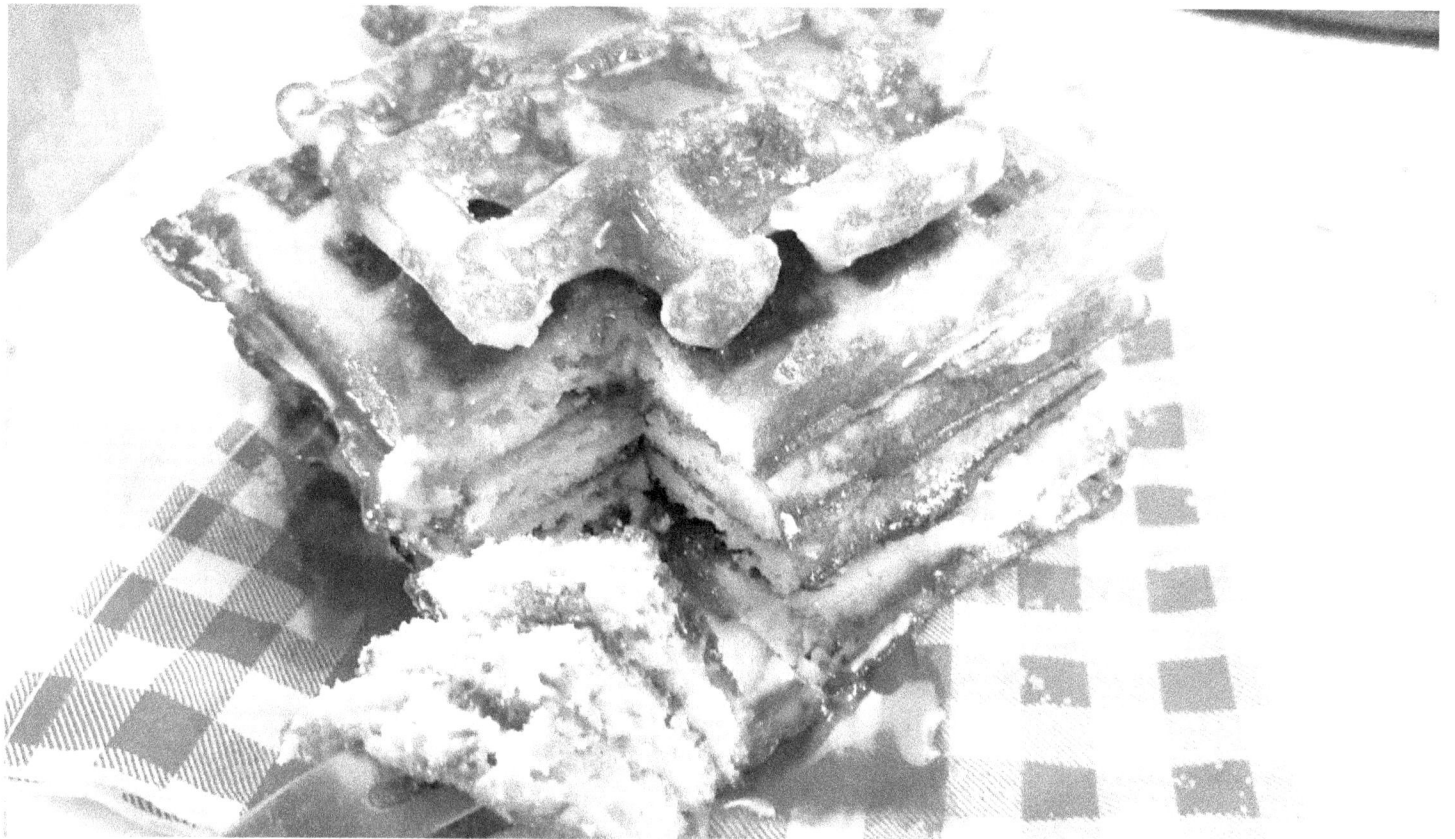

32 TASTY CHAFFLES

(Ready in about 13 minutes | Serving 2 | Difficulty: Easy)

Per serving: Kcal 116, Fat: 9.5gg, Net Carbs: 2.6g, Protein: 4.5g

Ingredients

- 1 oz softened cream cheese
- 1 tbsp of almond flour
- 1 tbsp of pumpkin puree
- 1 egg
- 1/2 tsp of pumpkin spice

Instructions

Whisk the cream cheese in a bowl. Whisk pumpkin puree and egg in a bowl. Add almond flour and pumpkin spice and mix. Preheat the iron and spray using oil. Pour half amount of mixture in the maker and cook for around 5 minutes. Repeat with the rest of the batter.

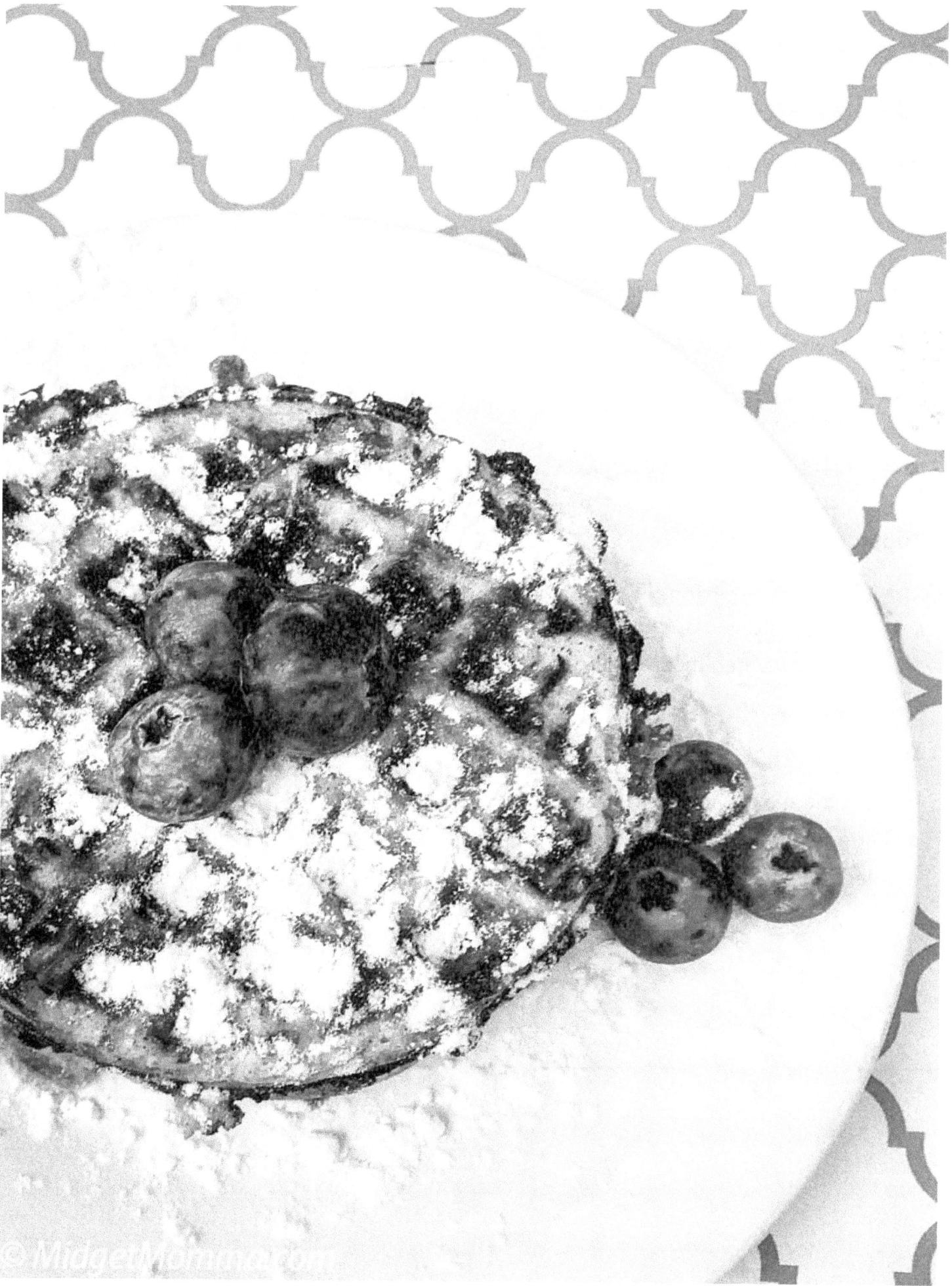

33 BREAD STICKS CHAFFLE

(Ready in about 12 minutes | Serving 7 | Difficulty: Easy)

Per serving: Kcal 80, Fat: 7g, Net Carbs: 1g, Protein: 5g

Ingredients

- 1 egg
- 2 tbsp of almond flour
- 1/2 cup grated mozzarella cheese
- 1/2tsp of garlic powder
- 1/2tsp of salt
- 1/2tsp of oregano

Topping

- 1/2tsp of garlic powder
- 2 tbsp softened butter
- 1/4 cup grated mozzarella cheese

Instructions

Preheat the maker and oil it. Mix all ingredients except topping ingredients. Pour in the maker and cook for around 5 minutes. Make four strips of waffle. Mix butter and garlic powder and coat strips with it. Sprinkle with mozzarella and cook for around 3 minutes.

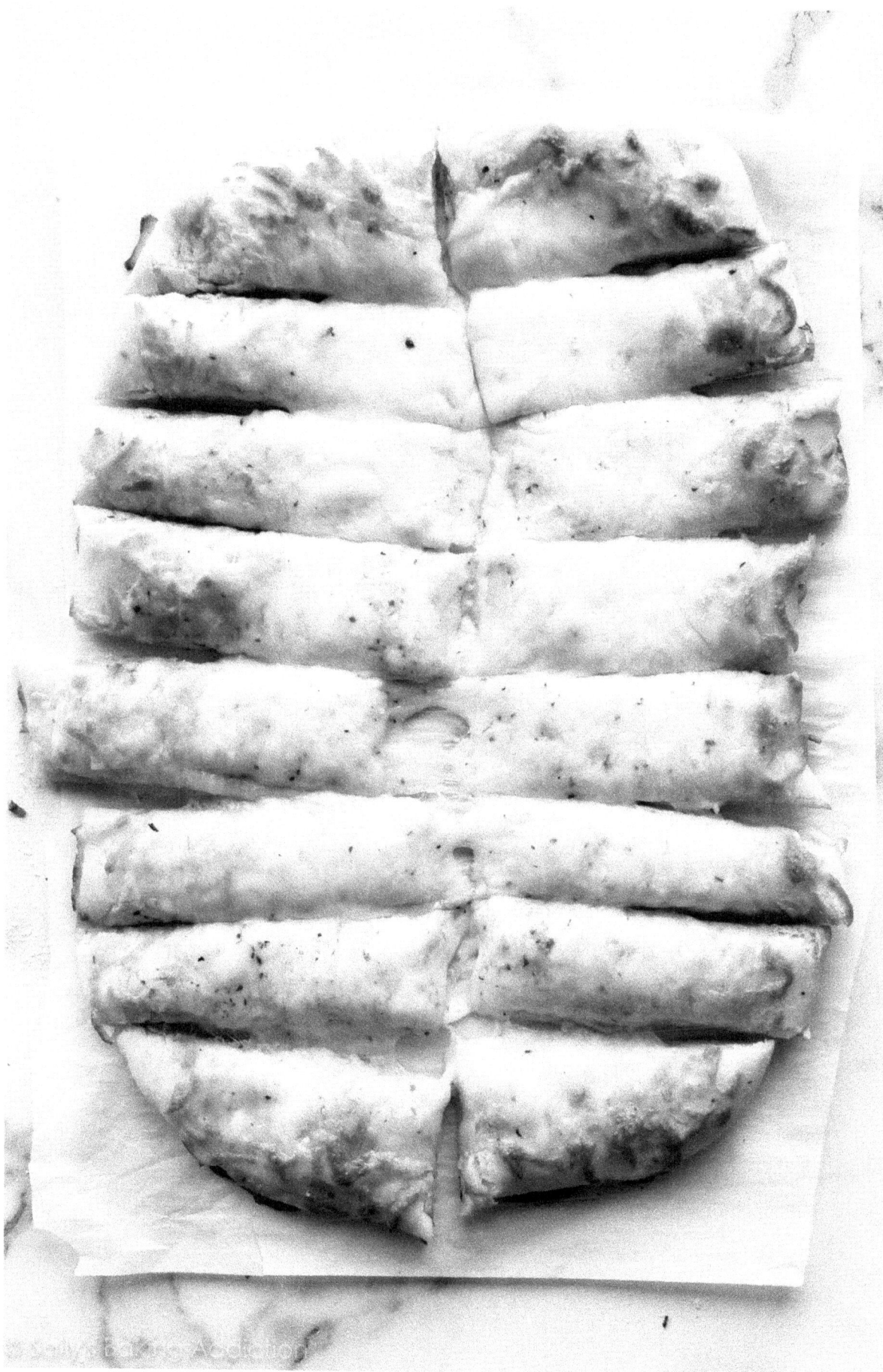

34 ORIGINAL CHAFFLE

(Ready in about 5 minutes | Serving 1 | Difficulty: Easy)

Per serving: Kcal 246, Fat: 18g, Net Carbs: 2g, Protein: 17g

Ingredients

- 2 eggs
- 1/4 cup of almond flour
- 1/2 cup of mozzarella
- 1/2 tsp of baking powder

Instructions

Preheat iron and spray with cooking spray. Mix all the ingredients in a bowl and pour half amount of the mixture into the maker. Cook for around 5 minutes and repeat with the rest of the mixture.

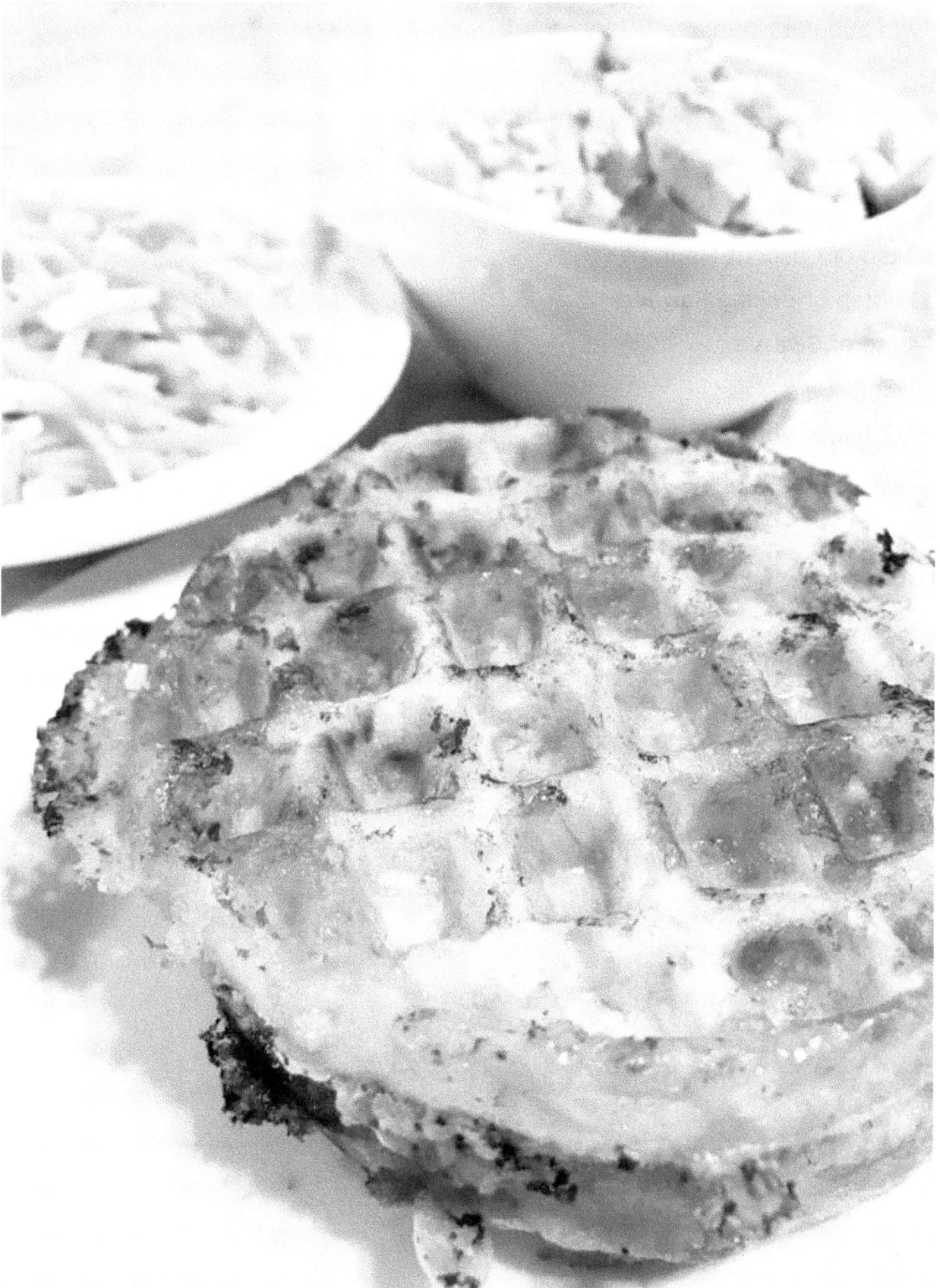

35 MINI CHAFFLES

(Ready in about 11 minutes | Serving 2 | Difficulty: Easy)

Per serving: Kcal 73, Fat: 6g, Net Carbs: 4g, Protein: 2g

Ingredients

- 2 tsp of Coconut Flour
- 1/4 tsp of Baking Powder
- 4 tsp of Swerve
- 1 Egg
- 1/2 tsp of Vanilla Extract
- 1 oz of Cream Cheese

Instructions

Preheat the iron. Add baking powder, coconut flour and swerve in a bowl and mix. Add cream cheese, egg and vanilla extract in bowl and mix. Pour mixture in the maker and cook for around 4 minutes.

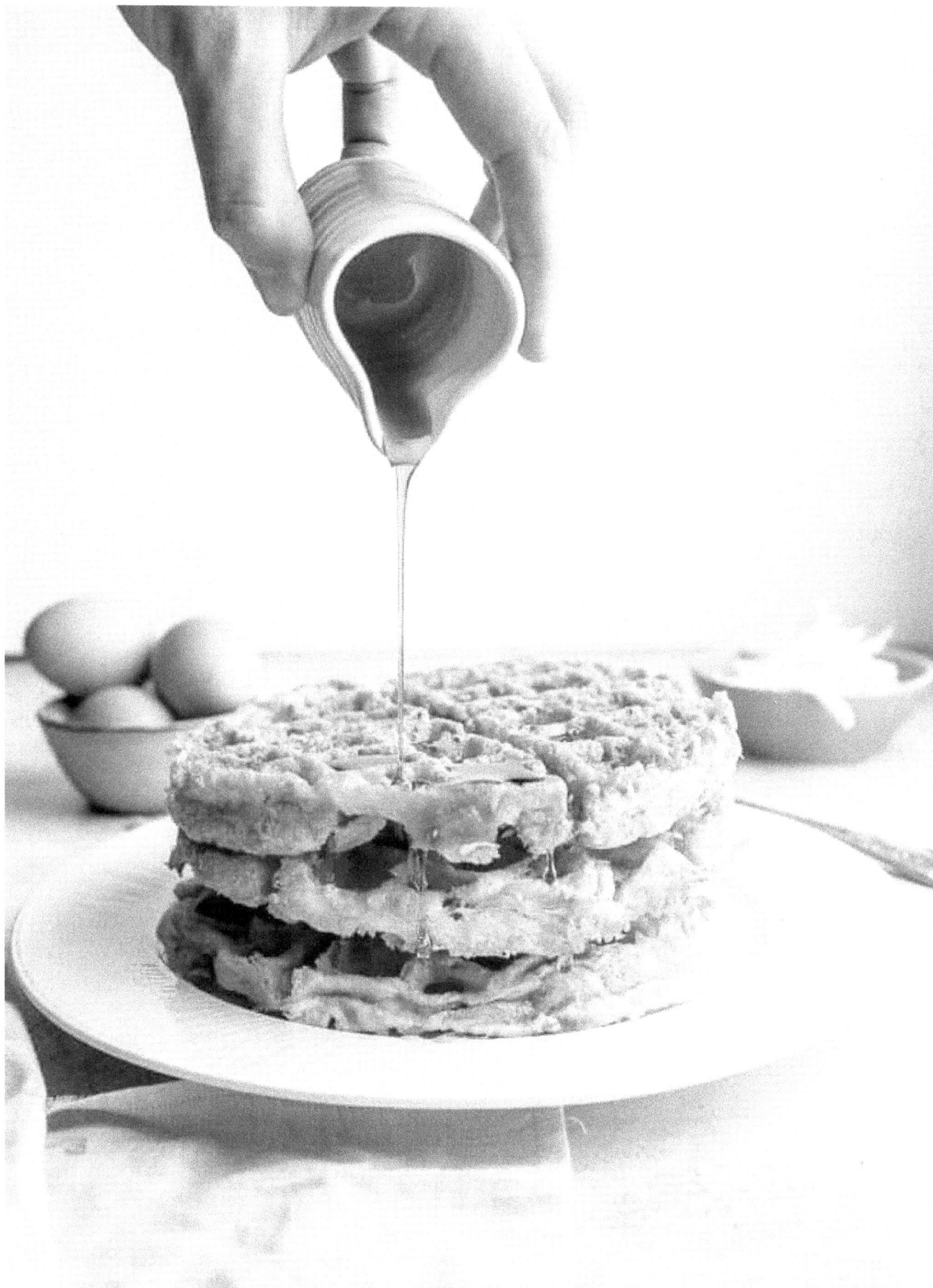

36 GRAIN-FREE CHAFFLES

(Ready in about 20 minutes | Serving 2 | Difficulty: Easy)

Per serving: Kcal 277, Fat: 20g, Net Carbs: 4.6g, Protein: 4.8g

Ingredients

- 1 tbsp of almond flour
- 1 tsp of vanilla
- 1 egg
- 1 shake of cinnamon
- 1 cup of mozzarella cheese
- 1 tsp of baking powder
- Butter

Instructions

Mix vanilla extract and egg in a bowl. Mix almond flour, baking powder and cinnamon. Add mozzarella cheese at the end and coat with the mixture evenly. Spray waffle using oil and turn it on. Pour mixture and cook for around 5 minutes. Top with butter and enjoy.

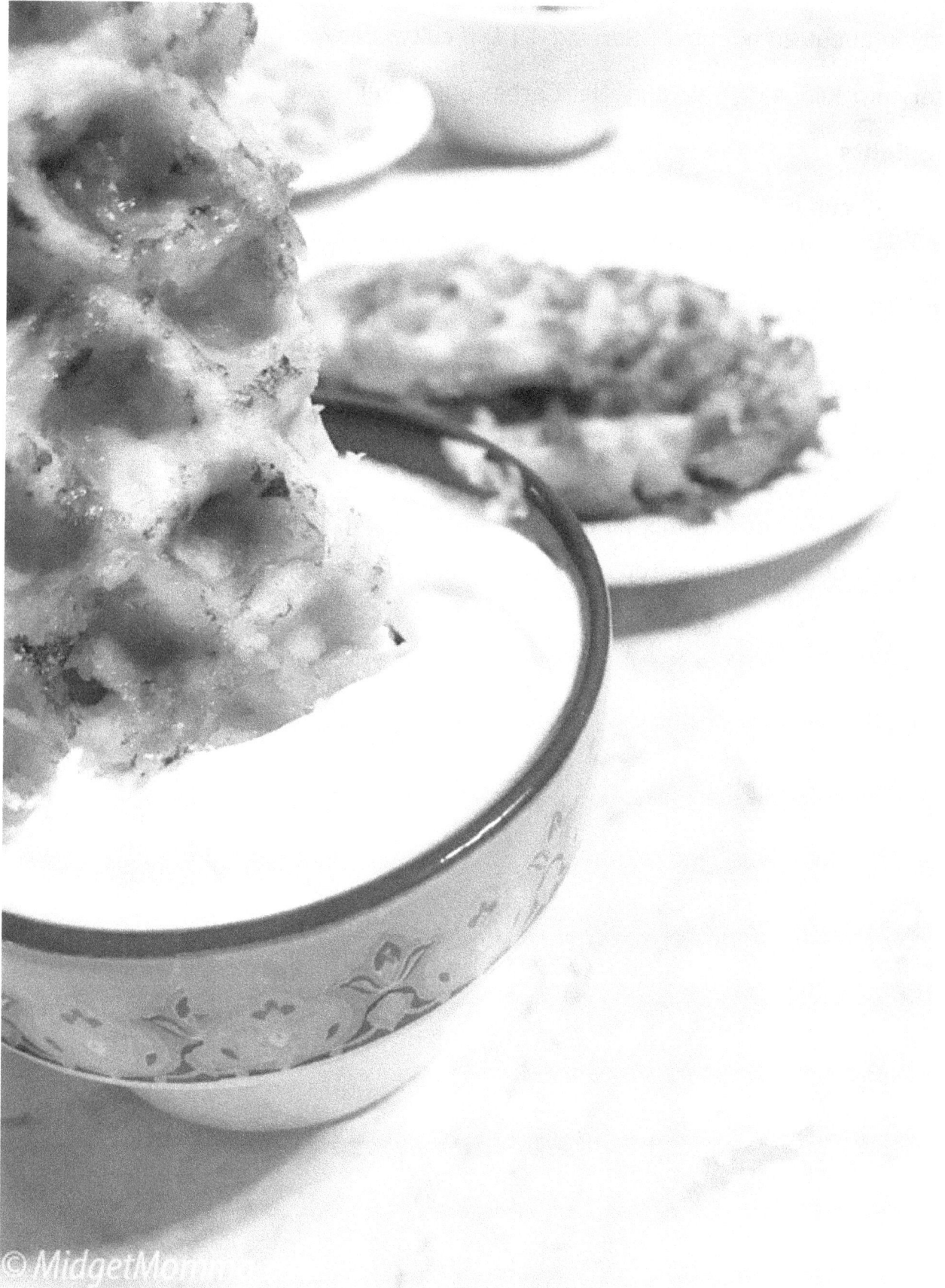

37 HEALTHY CHAFFLES

(Ready in about 20 minutes | Serving 4 | Difficulty: Easy)

Per serving: Kcal 411, Fat: 35g, Net Carbs: 6g, Protein: 21g

Ingredients

- 1 1/2 cup of shredded cheese cheddar
- 4 oz. cream cheese
- 4 eggs
- 2 tsp of baking powder
- 1/2 cup of almond flour
- Syrup

Instructions

Oil the waffle maker and mix all ingredients in a bowl. Pour batter into the maker and cook for around 5 minutes. Top with syrup(sugar-free) and enjoy.

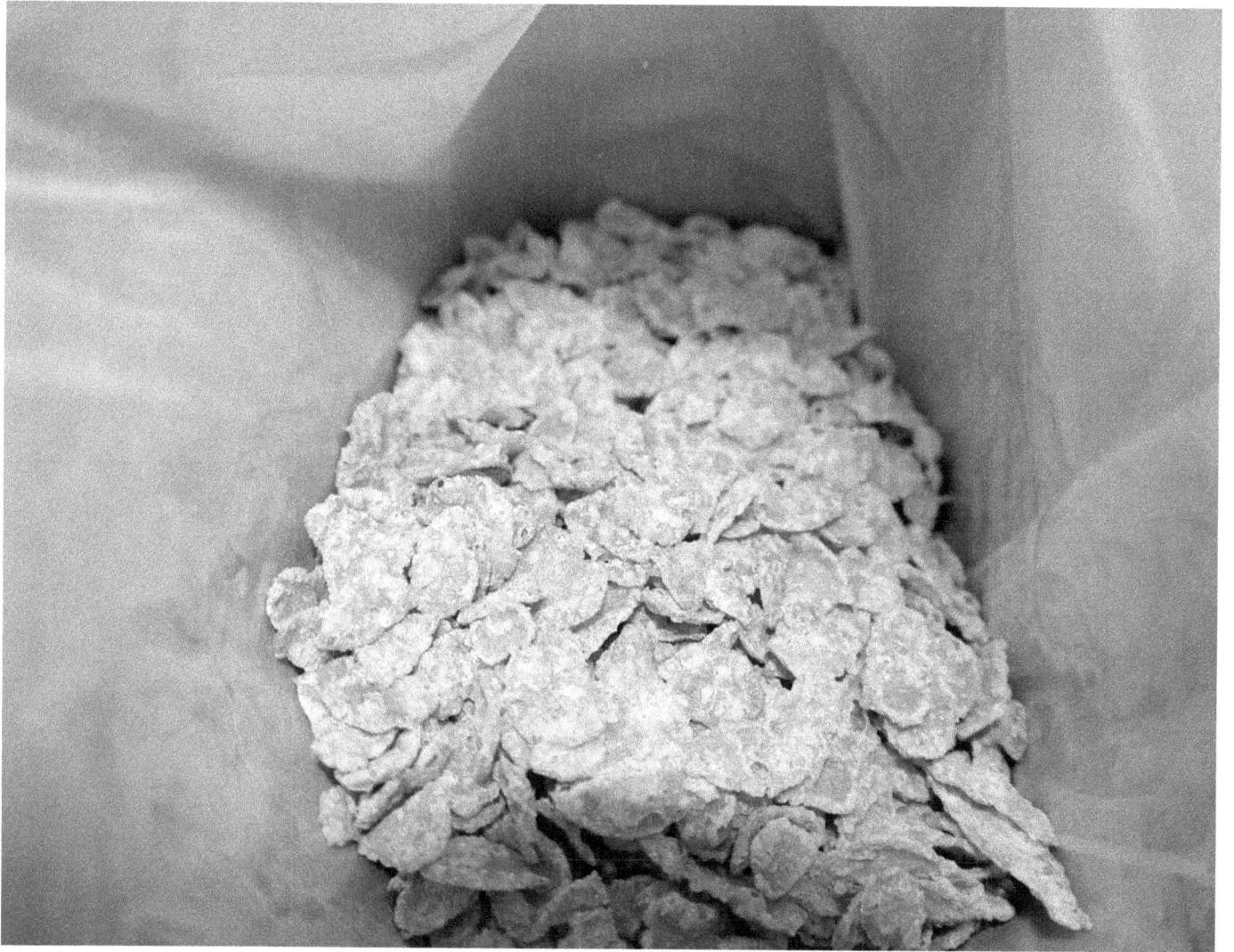

38 SUNNY CHAFFLE

(Ready in about 10 minutes | Serving 1 | Difficulty: Easy)

Per serving: Kcal 320, Fat: 24.3g, Net Carbs: 3.1g, Protein: 21.7g

Ingredients

- 1 egg
- Strawberries
- 2 tbsp of almond flour
- 1/2 cup of mozzarella cheese
- 1/2tsp of baking powder

Instructions

Preheat the maker and mix all the ingredients in a bowl. Pour into the center of the maker and cook for around 5 minutes. Top with strawberries and enjoy.

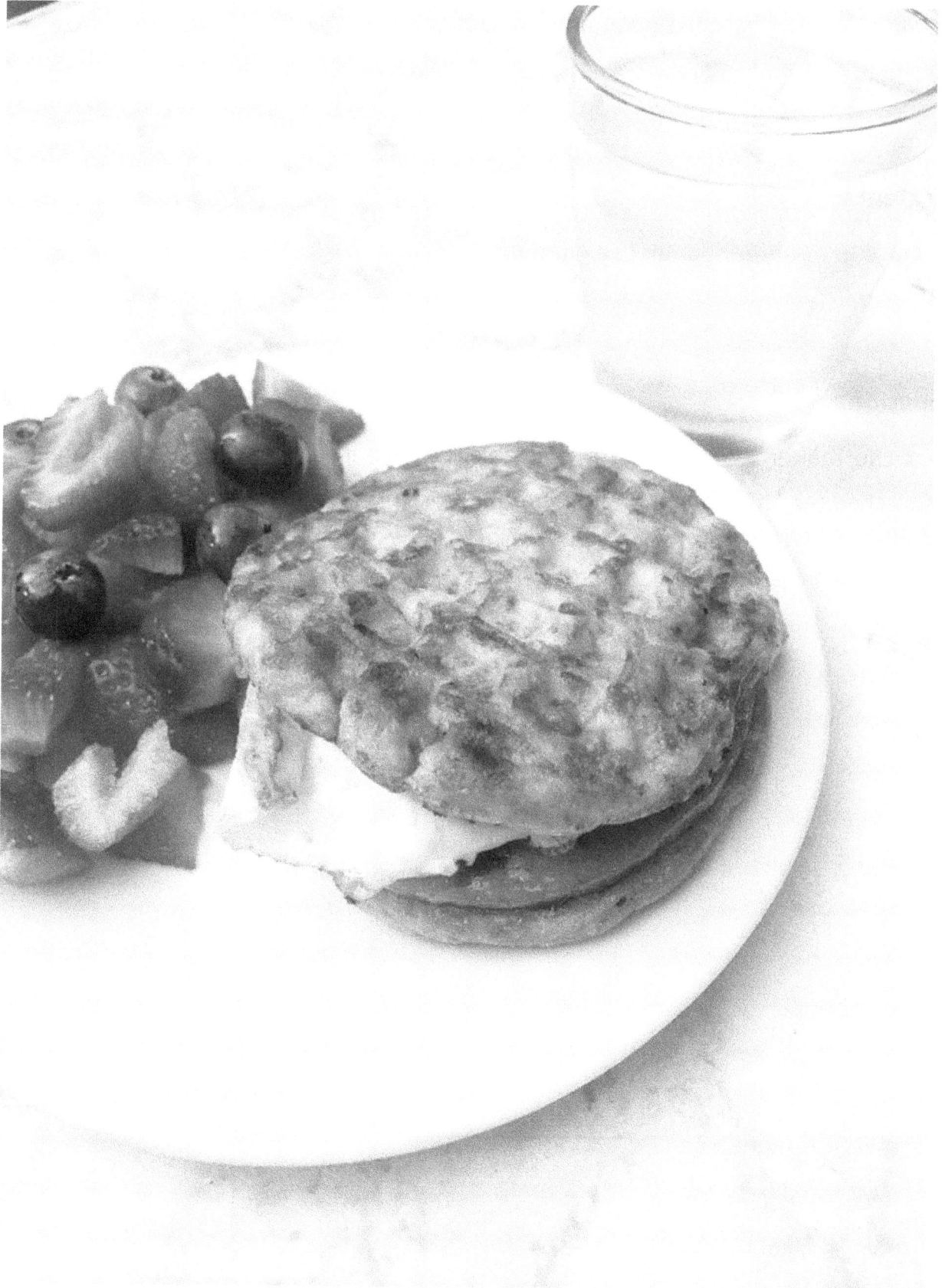

39 TRADITIONAL CHAFFLES

(Ready in about 13 minutes | Serving 1 | Difficulty: Easy)

Per serving: Kcal 291, Fat: 23g, Net Carbs: 1g, Protein: 20g

Ingredients

- 1/2 cup of shredded cheese cheddar
- 1 egg

Instructions

Preheat the maker and oil it gently. Break the egg in a bowl and add the half cup of cheddar cheese. Mix and pour half amount of mixture in maker. Cook for around 4 minutes. Repeat with the rest of the mixture.

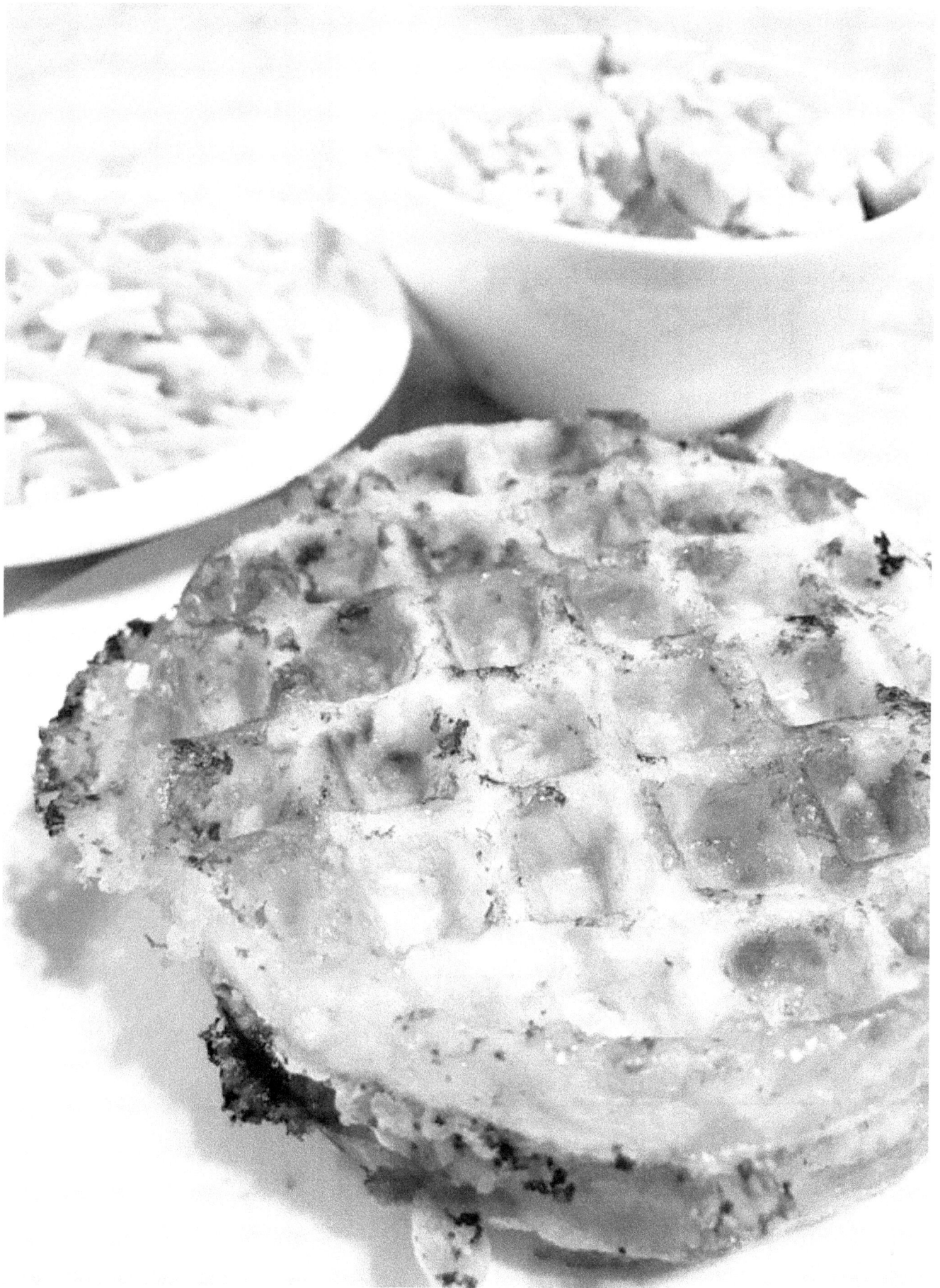

40 BEST PIZZA CHAFFLE

(Ready in about 20 minutes | Serving 2 | Difficulty: Easy)

Per serving: Kcal 241, Fat: 18g, Net Carbs: 4g, Protein: 17g

Ingredients

- 1 tsp of coconut flour
- 1/2 cup of shredded cheese mozzarella
- 1 white of egg
- `1 tsp softened cream cheese
- 1/8 tsp of Italian seasoning
- 1/4 tsp of baking powder
- 1/8 tsp of garlic powder
- 3 tsp of marinara sauce
- Salt
- 1/2 cup of mozzarella cheese
- 1 tbsp shredded cheese parmesan
- 6 pepperonis diced in half
- 1/4 tsp of basil seasoning

Instructions

Preheat the oven to 400 degrees F. Preheat the maker as well. Add all the ingredients except pepperoni and parmesan cheese in a bowl and mix. Pour half amount of mixture in the maker and cook for around 4 minutes. Repeat with the rest of the mixture. Top with pepperoni, tomato sauce and parmesan cheese. Bake in the oven by placing on the top shelf for around 6 minutes. Turn broil setting and cook for around 2 minutes. Sprinkle with basil.

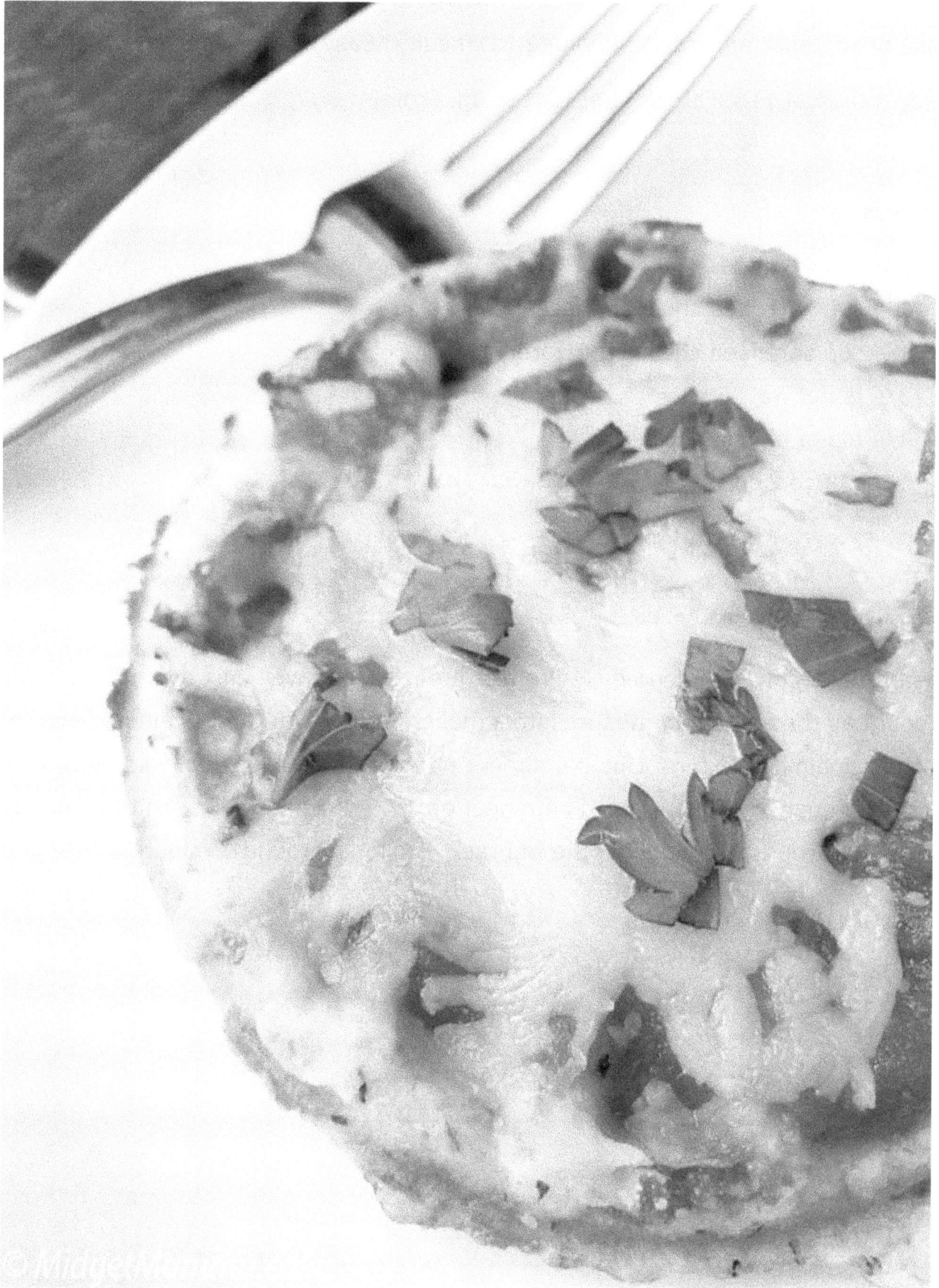

41 OPEN-FACED CHAFFLE

(Ready in about 17 minutes | Serving 2 | Difficulty: Easy)

Per serving: Kcal 118, Fat: 8g, Net Carbs: 2g, Protein: 9g

Ingredients

- 1 egg only white
- 1/4 cup shredded cheddar cheese
- 1/4 cup shredded cheese mozzarella
- 3/4 tsp of water
- 1/4 tsp of baking powder
- 1 tsp of coconut flour
- Salt

Instructions

Preheat the oven to 425 degrees F. Preheat the maker as well. Mix everything in a bowl and pour half the amount of mixture into a maker. Cook for around 4 minutes and repeat with the remaining mixture. Line parchment paper on a cookie sheet and place chaffles on it. Add a quarter cup of roasted keto beef gravy. Add cheese slice on top and bake in the oven for around 5 minutes in the top rack. Broil for around 1 minute.

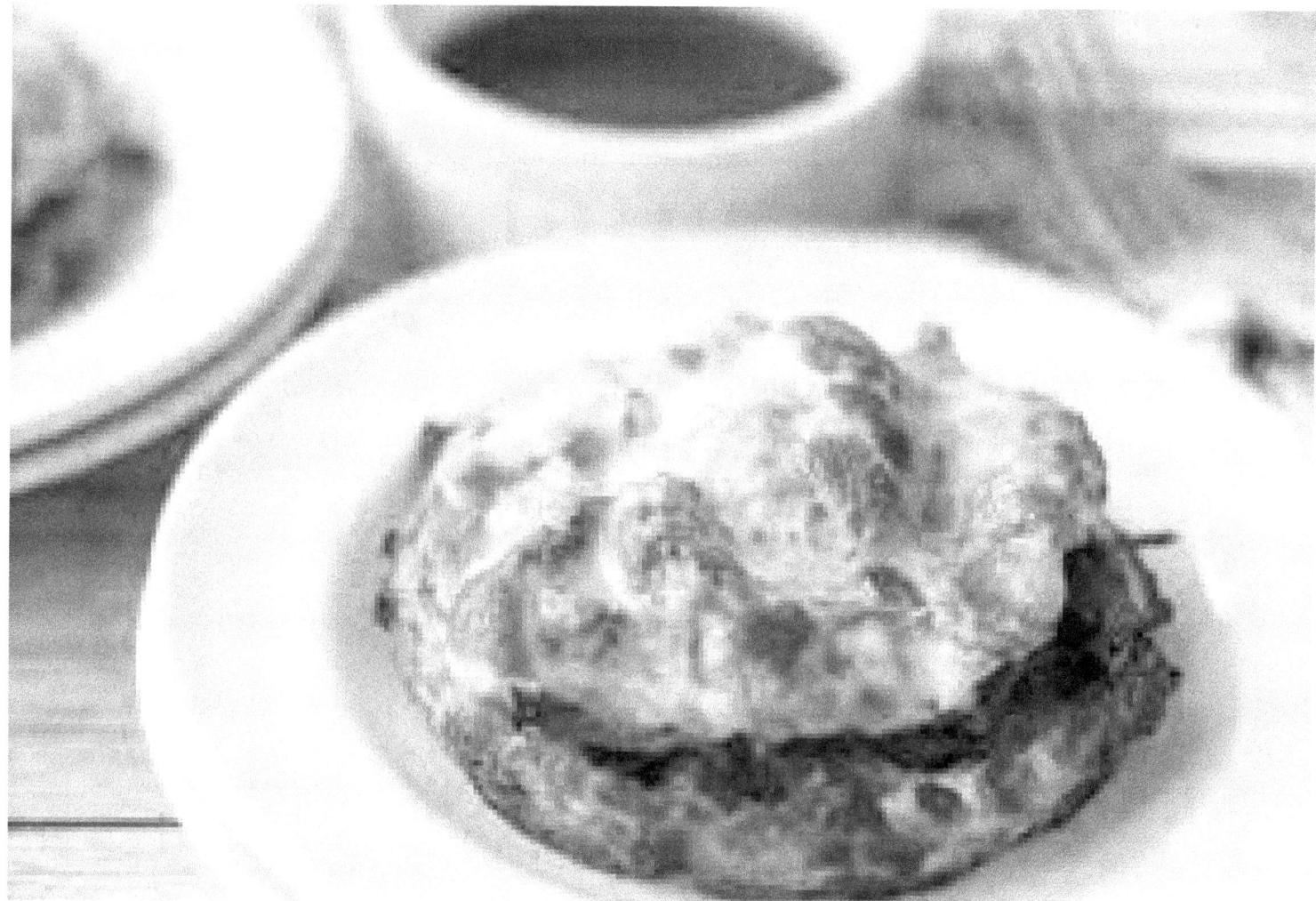

42 CREAM CHAFFLES

(Ready in about 15 minutes | Serving 2 | Difficulty: Easy)

Per serving: Kcal 293, Fat: 27g, Net Carbs: 5g, Protein: 10g

Ingredients

- 4 eggs
- 1 tsp of vanilla extract
- 2 tbsp of melted butter
- 4 oz of cream cheese
- 1 tsp of baking powder

Instructions

Blend all ingredients in a blender for around 1 minute. Spray the waffle maker using cooking spray and pour the mixture into the maker. Cook until it turns crispy and golden.

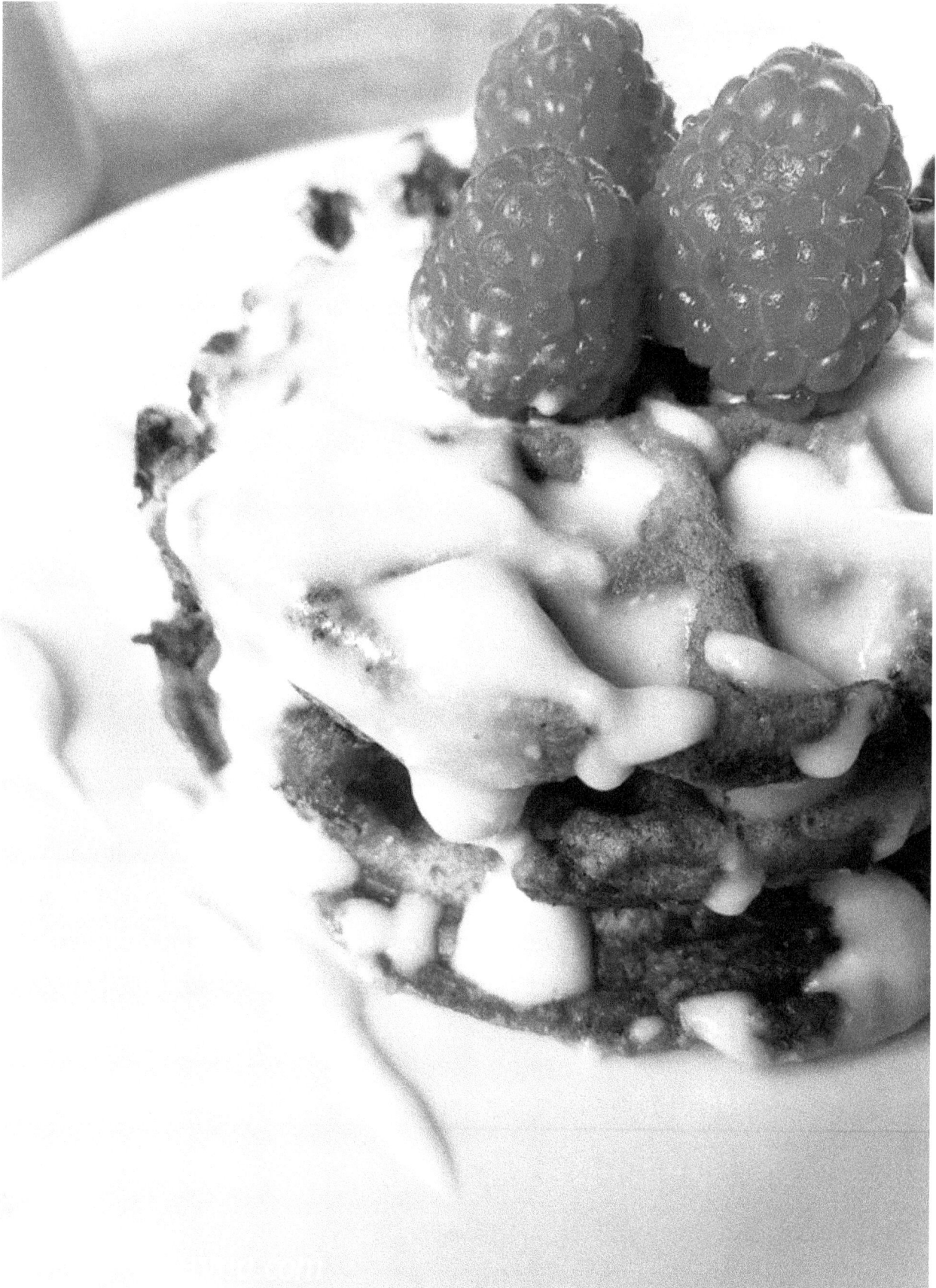

43 FLUFFY CHAFFLES

(Ready in about 45 minutes | Serving 8 | Difficulty: Moderate)

Per serving: Kcal 140, Fat: 11g, Net Carbs: 4g, Protein: 4g

Ingredients

- 64 g of almond flour
- 1 1/2 tsp of baking powder
- 1 tbsp of ground psyllium husk
- 28 g of coconut flour
- 1 tsp of xanthan gum
- 57 g of butter
- 240 ml of water
- 3 tbsp of erythritol
- 3 eggs beaten
- 1/4 tsp of kosher salt
- 1 tsp of vanilla extract

Instructions

Mix flours, xantham gum and husk in a bowl. Warm water, sweetener, salt and butter in a pot and once it starts simmering, add flours and incorporate. Cook for around 3 minutes. Transfer dough to bowl and add egg one by one, mixing using an electric mixer. Add baking powder and vanilla extract and mix. Heat the maker and oil it. Pour batter and cook for around 12 minutes.

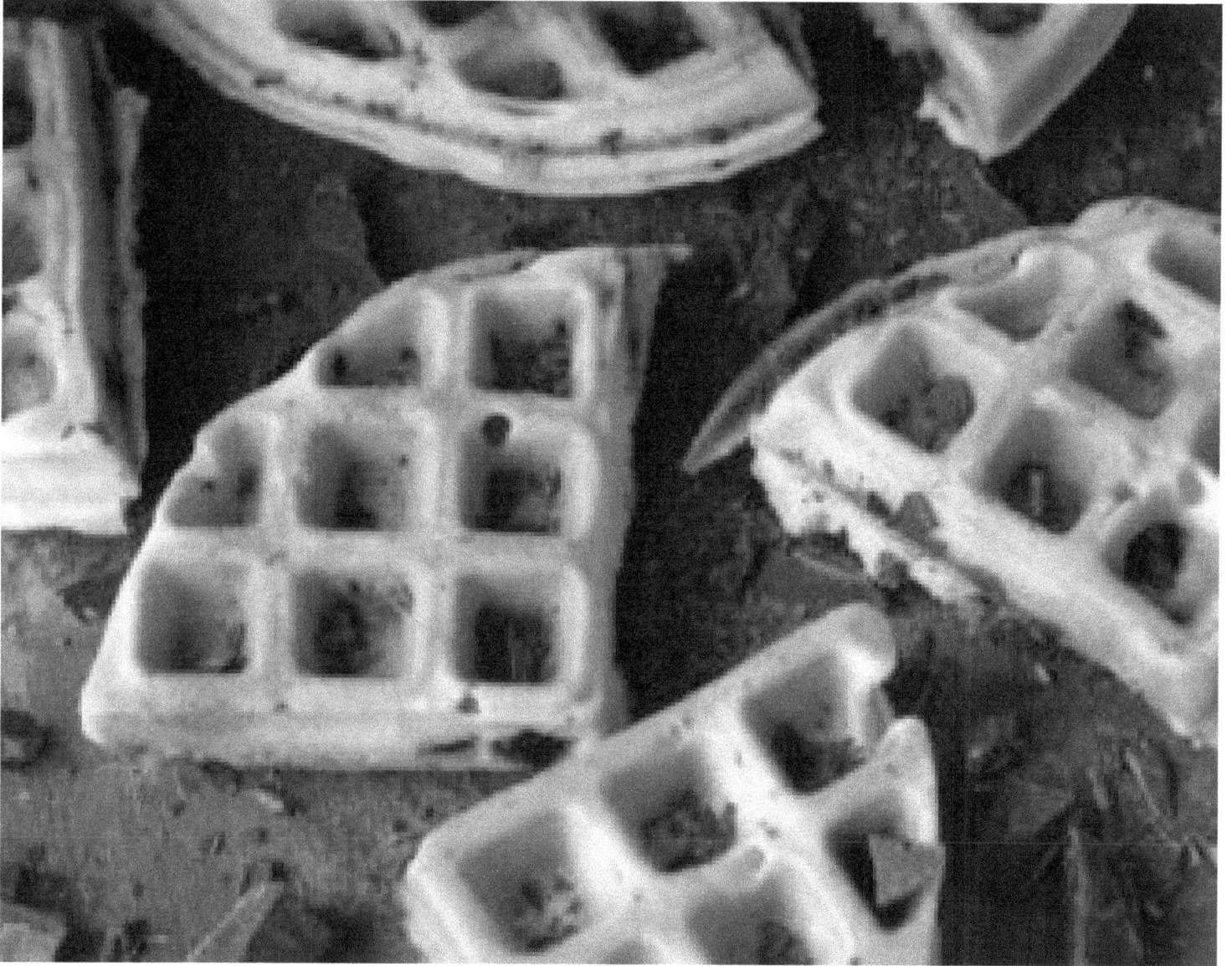

44 ALMOND FLOUR CHAFFLES

(Ready in about 20 minutes | Serving 2 | Difficulty: Easy)

Per serving: Kcal 70, Fat: 3.8g, Net Carbs: 4.9g, Protein: 4g

Ingredients

- 4 separated eggs
- 1/4 cup of granulated Swerve
- 2 cup of almond flour
- 2 tsp of baking powder
- 1/2 cup of butter
- 1 tsp of kosher salt
- 1/2 cup of almond butter
- Cooking spray
- 2 tsp. of vanilla extract
- Maple syrup

Instructions

Preheat waffle maker to high. Mix stevia, almond flour, salt and baking powder in a bowl. Melt almond butter and butter in the microwave for around 15 seconds. Stir dry ingredients with butter mixture and then add vanilla and yolks. Beat whites in a separate bowl and fold in batter. Spray maker using cooking spray and pour the batter. Cook for around 5 minutes. Top with maple syrup and butter.

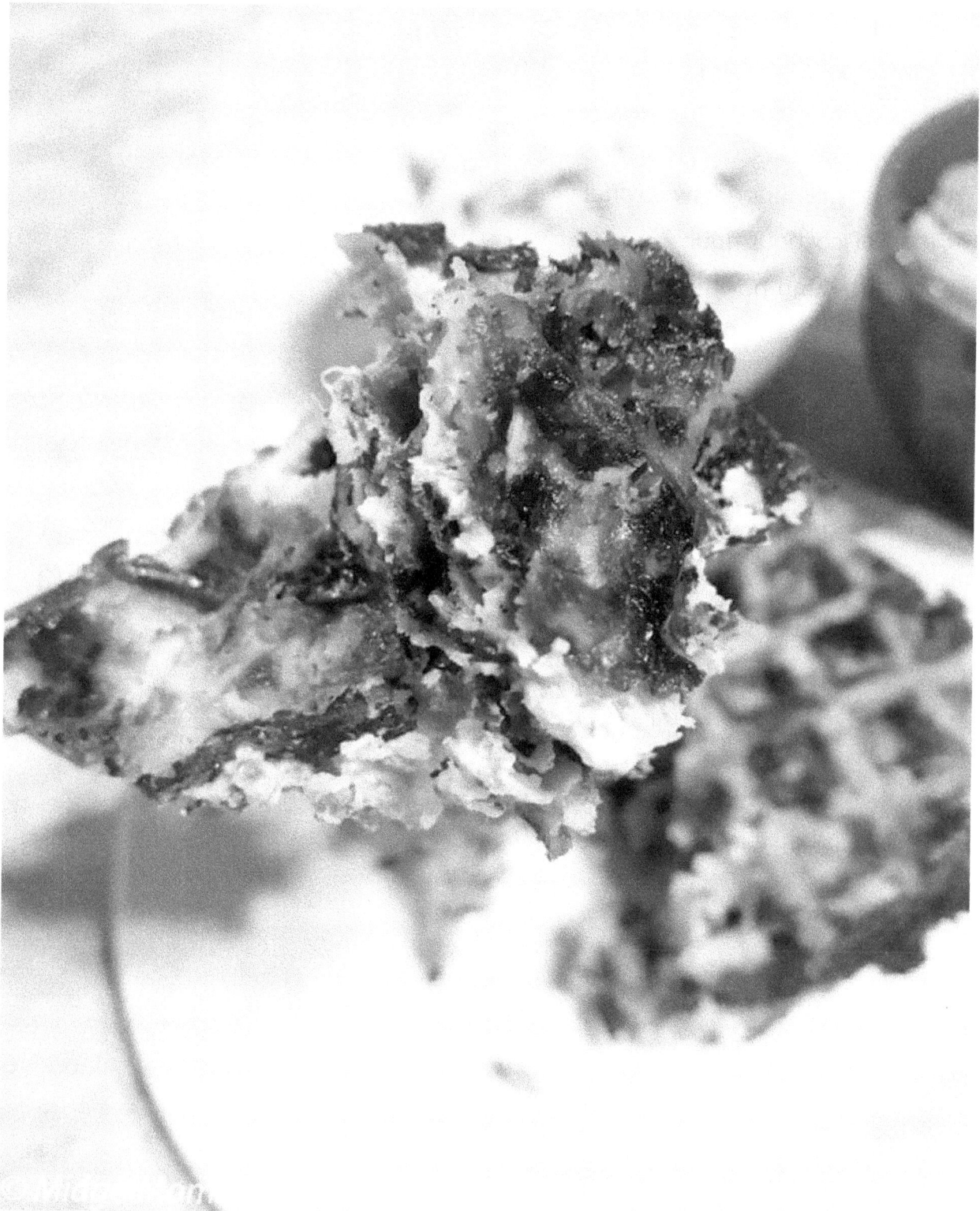

45 BUTTER CHAFFLES

(Ready in about 30 minutes | Serving 5 | Difficulty: Easy)

Per serving: Kcal 216, Fat: 19.9g, Net Carbs: 5.5g, Protein: 6.4g

Ingredients

- 5 eggs
- 4 tbsp of granulated sweetener
- 4 tbsp of coconut flour
- 1 tsp of baking powder
- 3 tbsp of milk full fat
- 2 tsp of vanilla
- 125 g of butter melted

Instructions

Beat egg whites in a bowl. Mix yolks with sweetener, baking powder and coconut flour in a separate bowl. Add butter and mix. Add vanilla and milk and mix. Fold whites in yolk mixture and pour in maker. Cook for around 5 minutes.

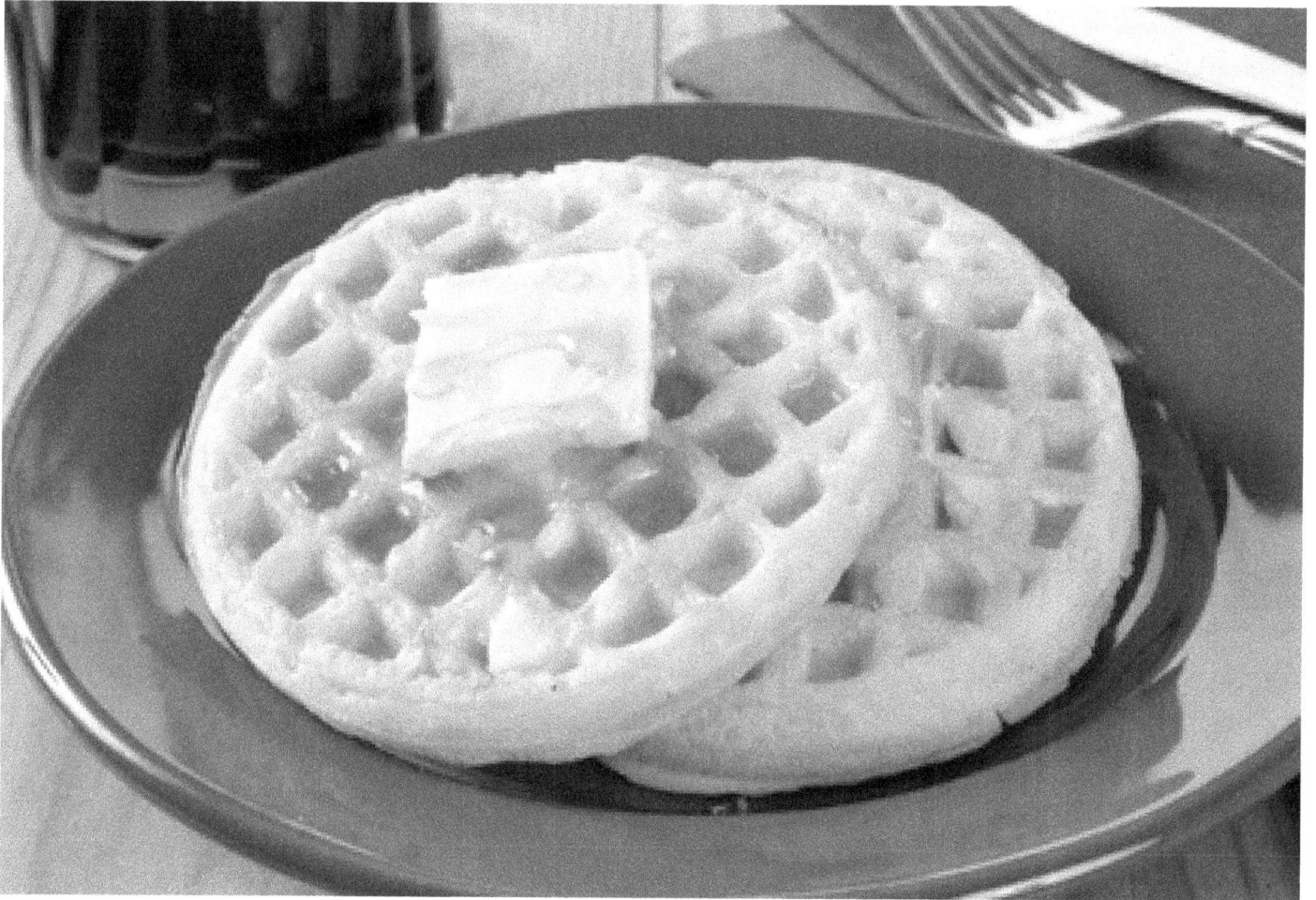

46 PALEO CHAFFLES

(Ready in about 10minutes | Serving 2 | Difficulty: Easy)

Per serving: Kcal 401, Fat: 37, Net Carbs: 9g, Protein: 13g

Ingredients

- 1 egg
- 2 tbsp of sweetener
- 1/2 cup of Almond Flour
- 1/2 tsp of baking powder Gluten-free
- 2 tbsp of Almond butter
- 1/4 tsp of Sea salt
- 2 tbsp of Butter
- 1/2 tsp of Vanilla extract
- 1/4 cup of almond milk Unsweetened

Instructions

Preheat waffle maker to high temperature. Oil it gently and beat whites in a bowl. Combine baking powder, erythritol, salt and almond flour in another bowl. Melt almond butter and butter in the microwave and add to the flour mixture. Add yolk, vanilla and almond milk and stir. Fold whites in batter and mix. Pour in the maker and cook for around 5 minutes.

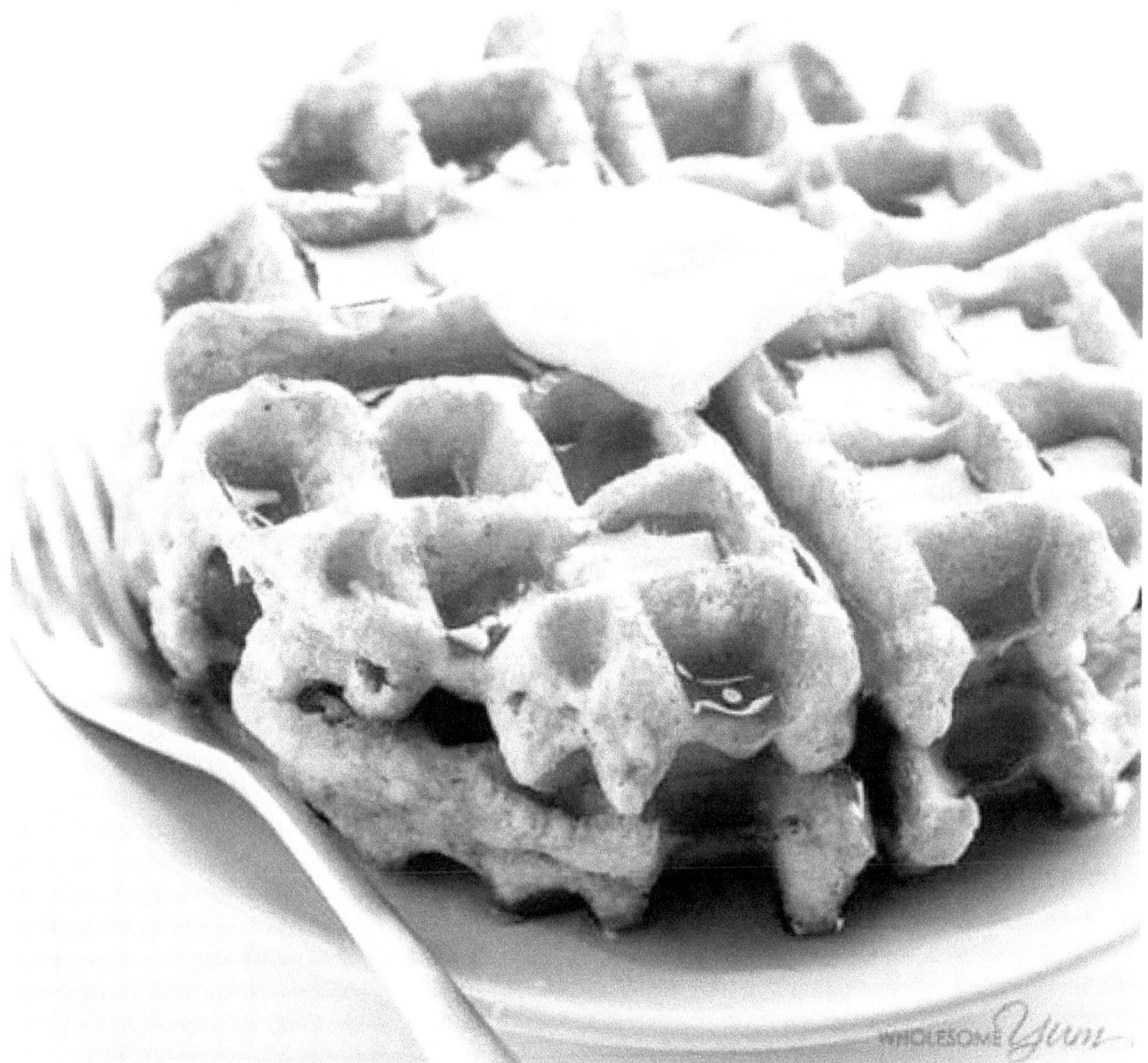

WHOLESOME *Yum*

47 CRISPY CHAFFLES

(Ready in about 10 minutes | Serving 4 | Difficulty: Easy)

Per serving: Kcal 64, Fat: 2g, Net Carbs: 4g, Protein: 5g

Ingredients

- 4 tbsp sifted coconut flour
- 1/4 tsp of baking powder
- 1 tsp of coconut oil
- 1 tbsp sweetener granulated
- 2/3 cup of egg whites
- 1/2 tsp of vanilla extract
- 1/4 cup of milk
- 1 tbsp of unsweetened apple sauce

Instructions

Mix sweetener, baking powder and coconut flour in a bowl. Add whites, vanilla, apple sauce and milk in a separate bowl and mix. Pour to the other bowl and form a thick batter. Add oil and spray waffle maker using cooking spray. Once the maker is hot, pour the batter and cook for around 4 minutes.

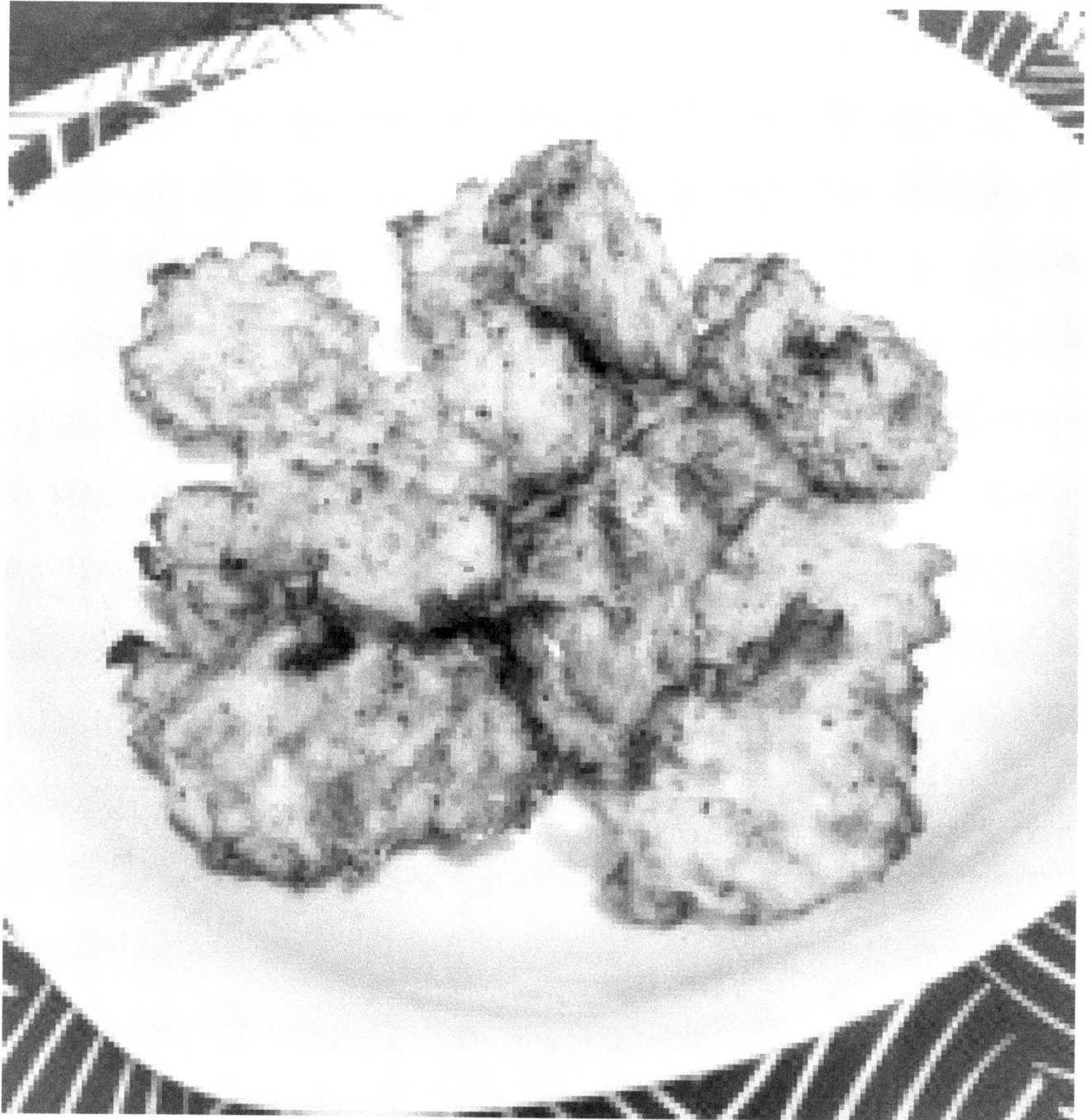

48 SALTED CHAFFLES

(Ready in about 15 minutes | Serving 2 | Difficulty: Easy)

Per serving: Kcal 425, Fat: 36.7g, Net Carbs: 10.7g, Protein: 14.8g

Ingredients

Dry

- 3/4 cup of Almond Flour
- 1 tbsp of Coconut flour
- 2 tbsp of Erythritol
- 1 tsp of Baking Powder
- 1/8 tsp of Himalayan Salt

Wet

- 2 tbsp of Melted Butter
- 2 Eggs
- 2 tbsp of Cream Cheese at room temperature
- 1 tsp of Vanilla Extract

Instructions

Preheat waffle maker to high. Mix wet ingredients in a bowl. Mix dry ingredients in a separate bowl. Mix both bowls and pour in the maker. Cook for around 4 minutes.

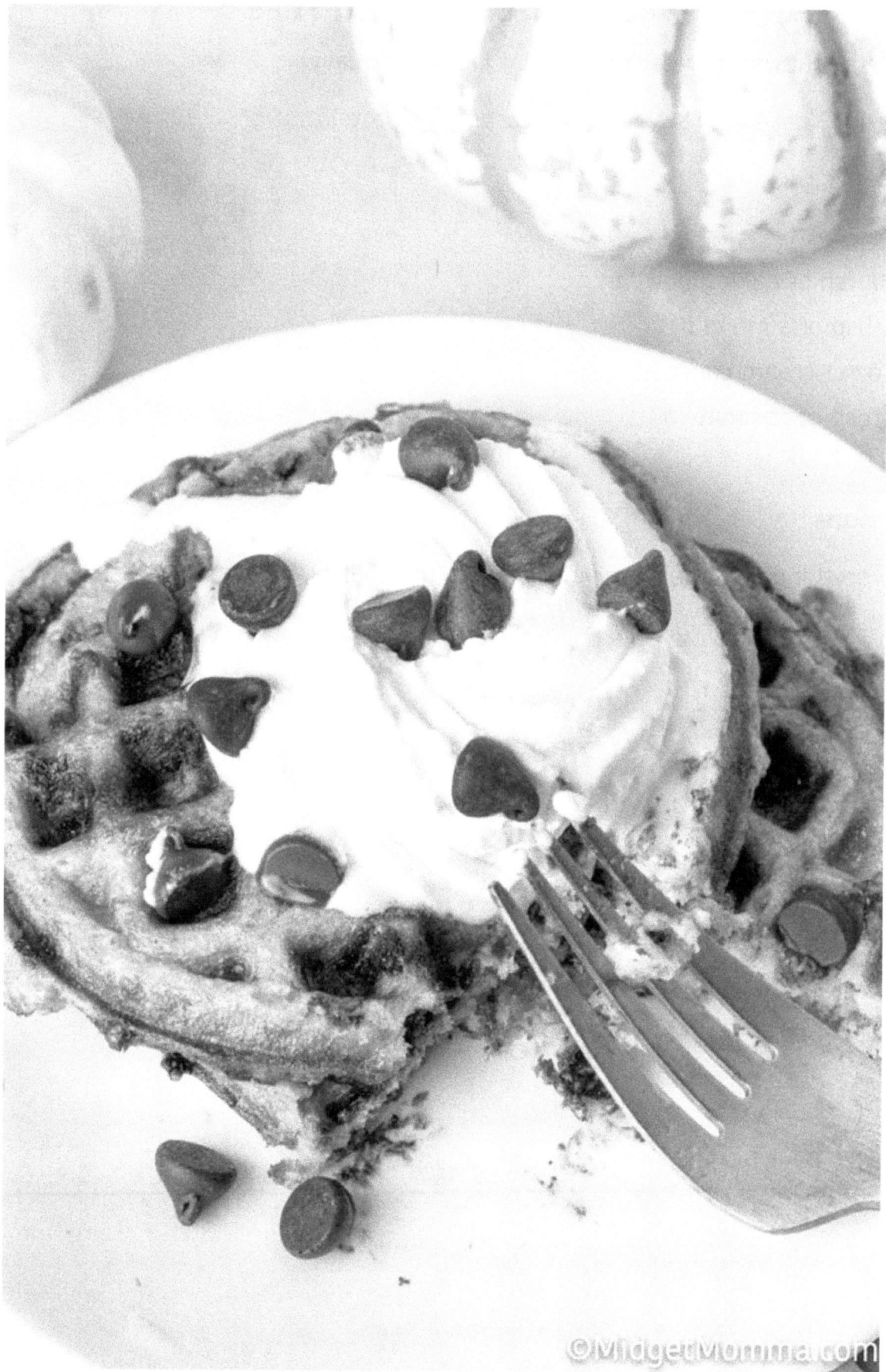

49 LOW CARB CHAFFLES

(Ready in about 8 minutes | Serving 1 | Difficulty: Easy)

Per serving: Kcal 522, Fat: 48g, Net Carbs: 7g, Protein: 19g

Ingredients

- 2 eggs
- 1/2 tsp of baking powder
- 4 tbsp of almond flour
- 2 oz of cream cheese
- 1 tbsp of coconut oil

Instructions

Blend everything in the blender and pour in the maker, which is oiled. Cook for around 3 minutes.

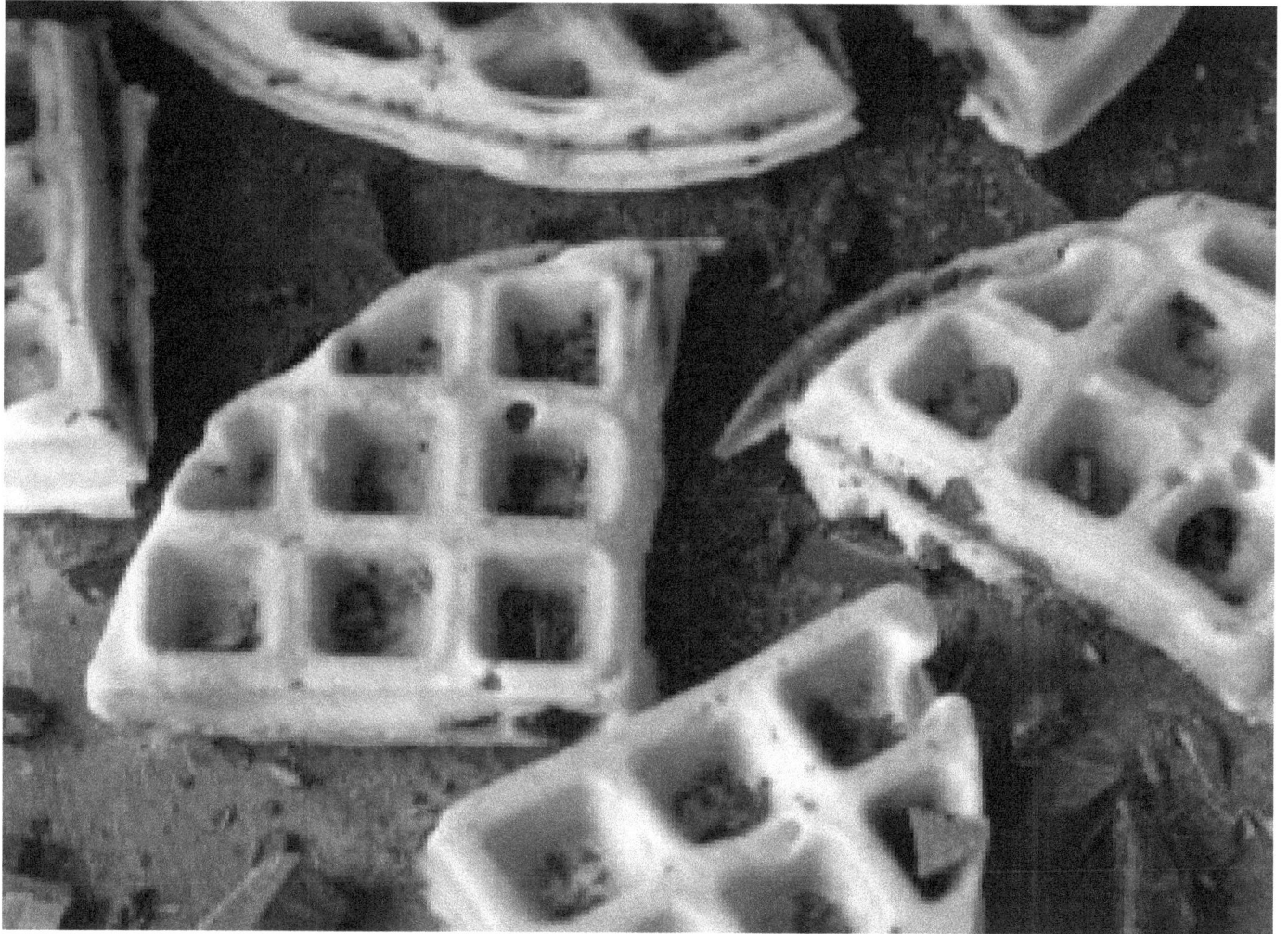

50 SWEET CHAFFLES

(Ready in about 9 minutes | Serving 2 | Difficulty: Easy)

Per serving: Kcal 331, Fat: 29g, Net Carbs: 7g, Protein: 11g

Ingredients

Dry

- 1/2 cup of almond flour
- 1/2 tsp of sweetener
- 1/4tsp of baking soda
- 1/4tsp of salt
- 1/4 tsp of baking powder
- 1/8 tsp of nutmeg
- 1/4tsp of ground cinnamon
- 1/8 tsp of cloves

Wet

- 2 eggs
- 2 tbsp of melted butter
- 1 tsp of vanilla extract

Instructions

Add dry ingredients to a bowl and mix. Separate yolks and whites in two bowls and mix butter and vanilla in yolks. Beat whites and add yolks to dry ingredients. Then add whites while mixing gently. Preheat maker to high temperature and pour the mixture. Cook for around 5 minutes.

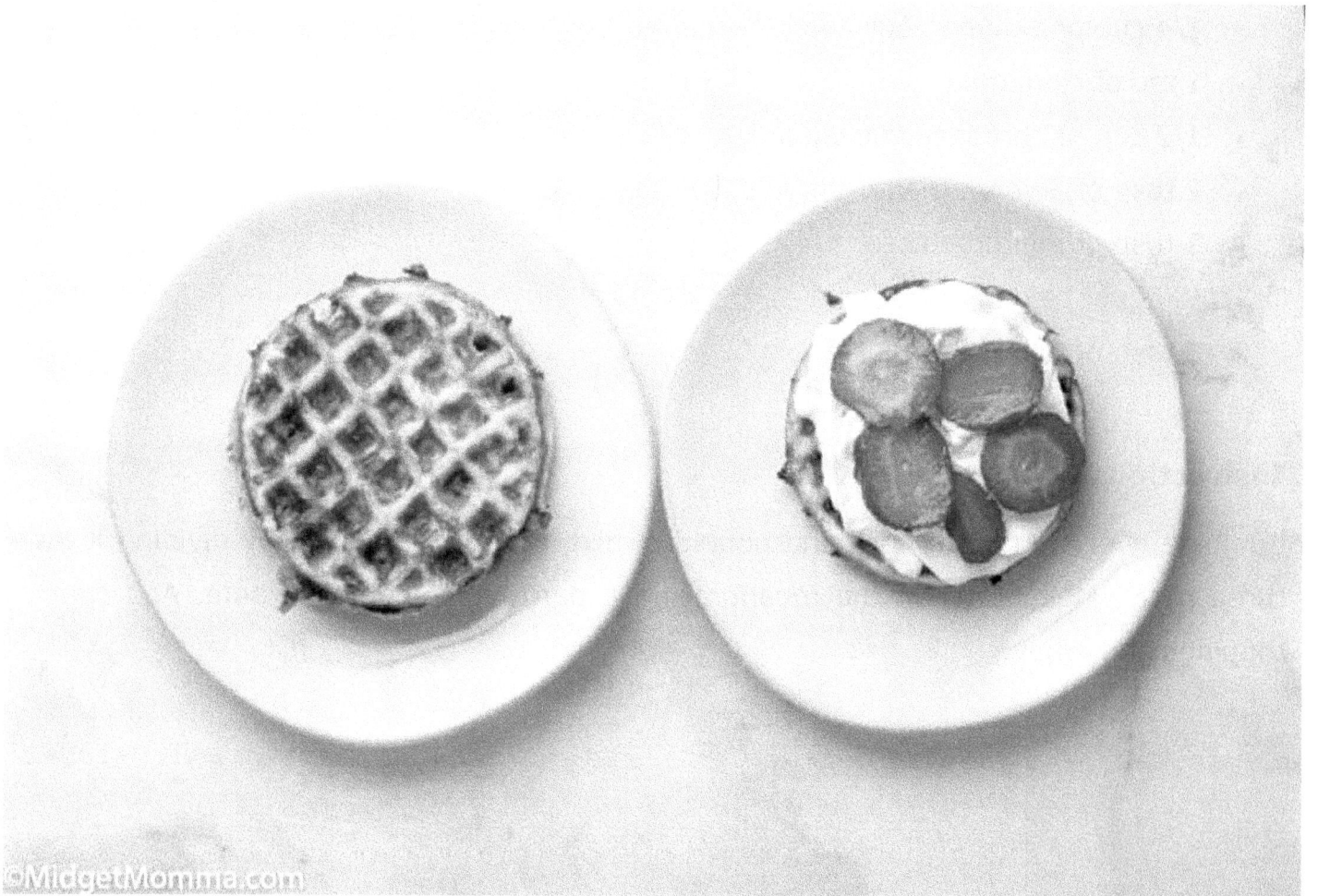

51 CHURRO CHAFFLE

(Ready in about 15 minutes | Serving 1 | Difficulty: Easy)

Per serving: Kcal 193, Fat: 14g, Net Carbs: 2g, Protein: 8g

Ingredients

- 1 egg
- 1/4 cup of almond flour
- 1 tsp of cinnamon
- 1/2 cup of shredded cheese mozzarella
- 2 tbsp of Swerve granular
- 2 tbsp of melted butter
- ⅛ tsp of baking powder
- 3 tbsp of Swerve granular

Instructions

Combine everything in a bowl and pour the mixture into the maker by dividing it into three parts. Melt butter in the meantime in a pan over moderate flame. Add churro toppings and enjoy.

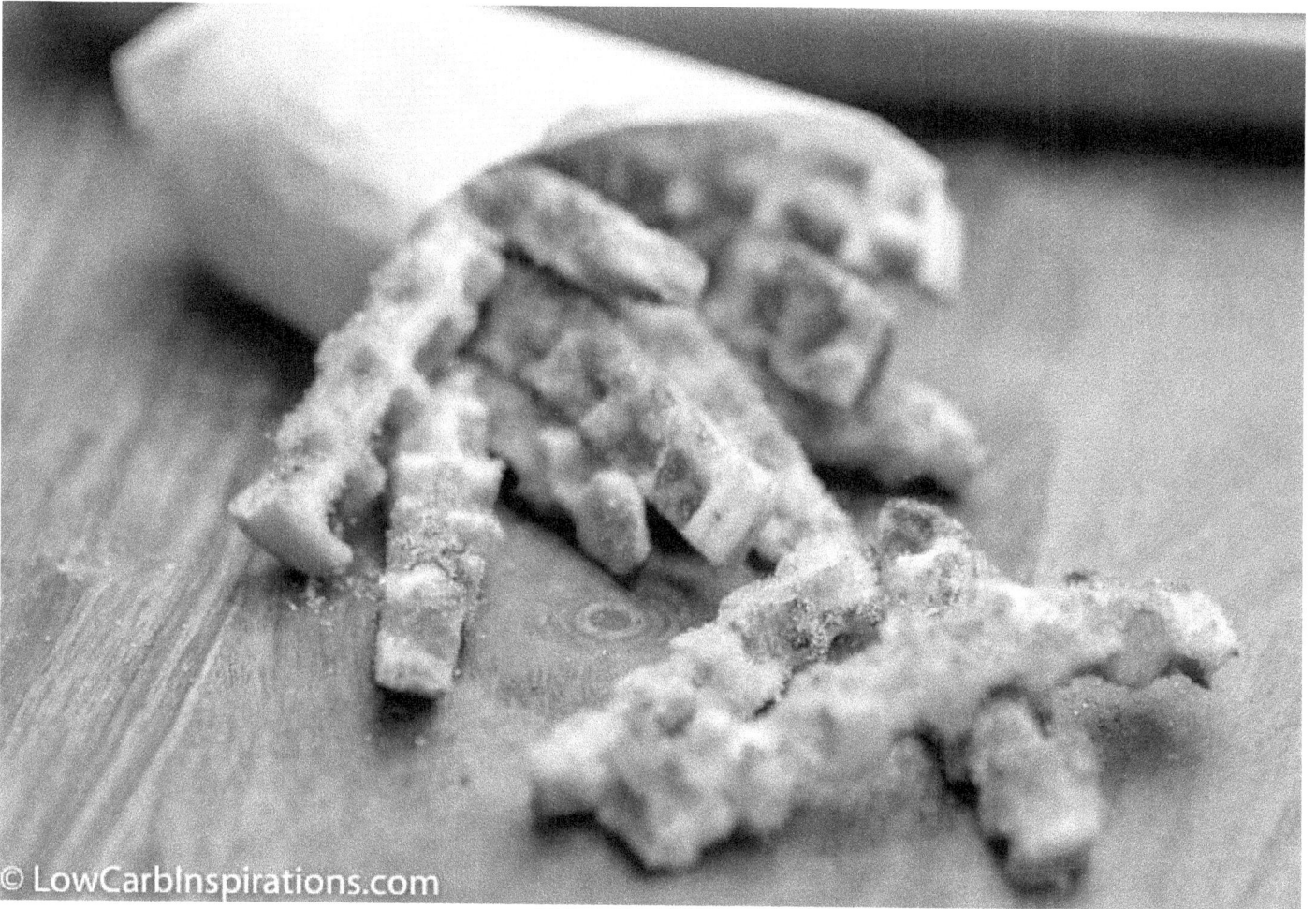

52 AVOCADO EGG BAKE

(Ready in about 20 minutes | Serving 1 | Difficulty: Easy)

Per serving: Kcal 605, Fat: 50.9g, Net Carbs: 18.6g, Protein: 25.3g

Ingredients

- 2 eggs
- 1 avocado, pitted and halved
- ¼ cup of shredded Cheddar cheese
- 1 tbsp. chopped fresh parsley, or according to taste
- Freshly ground black pepper and salt according to taste

Instructions

- Preheat oven to 425 degrees Fahrenheit.
- To make way for one egg, scoop out some of the avocados from where the pit. Put each avocado half on the baking sheet, then crack one egg on top.
- Cook for fifteen to twenty minutes in a preheated oven before the egg is ready. Season with pepper and salt and finish with Cheddar cheese. Serve with new parsley as a garnish.

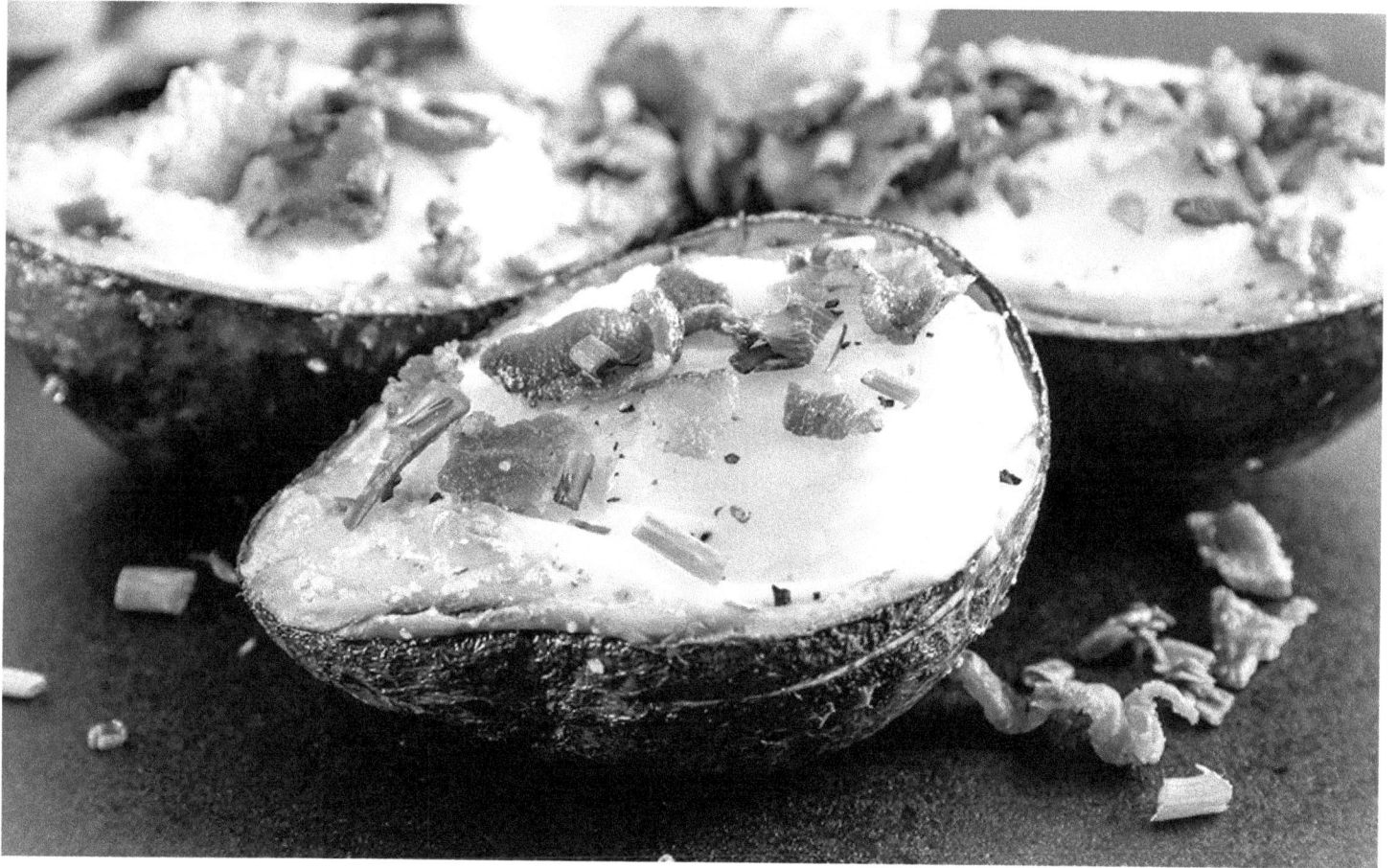

53 OVEN-BAKED BACON

(Ready in about 35 minutes | Serving 6 | Difficulty: Easy)

Per serving: Kcal 134, Fat: 10.4g, Net Carbs: 0.4g, Protein: 9.2g

Ingredients

1 (16 oz.) package bacon

Instructions

- Preheat oven to 350°F. Using parchment paper, line a baking dish.
- Put the bacon slices on a prepared baking sheet, one on top of the other.
- Bake for fifteen to twenty minutes in a preheated oven. Take off the dish from the oven. Return the bacon slices to the oven after tossing them with kitchen tongs. Bake for another fifteen to twenty minutes, or till crispy. Thinner slices may require less time to cook, about twenty minutes overall. Drain on a paper towel-lined pan.

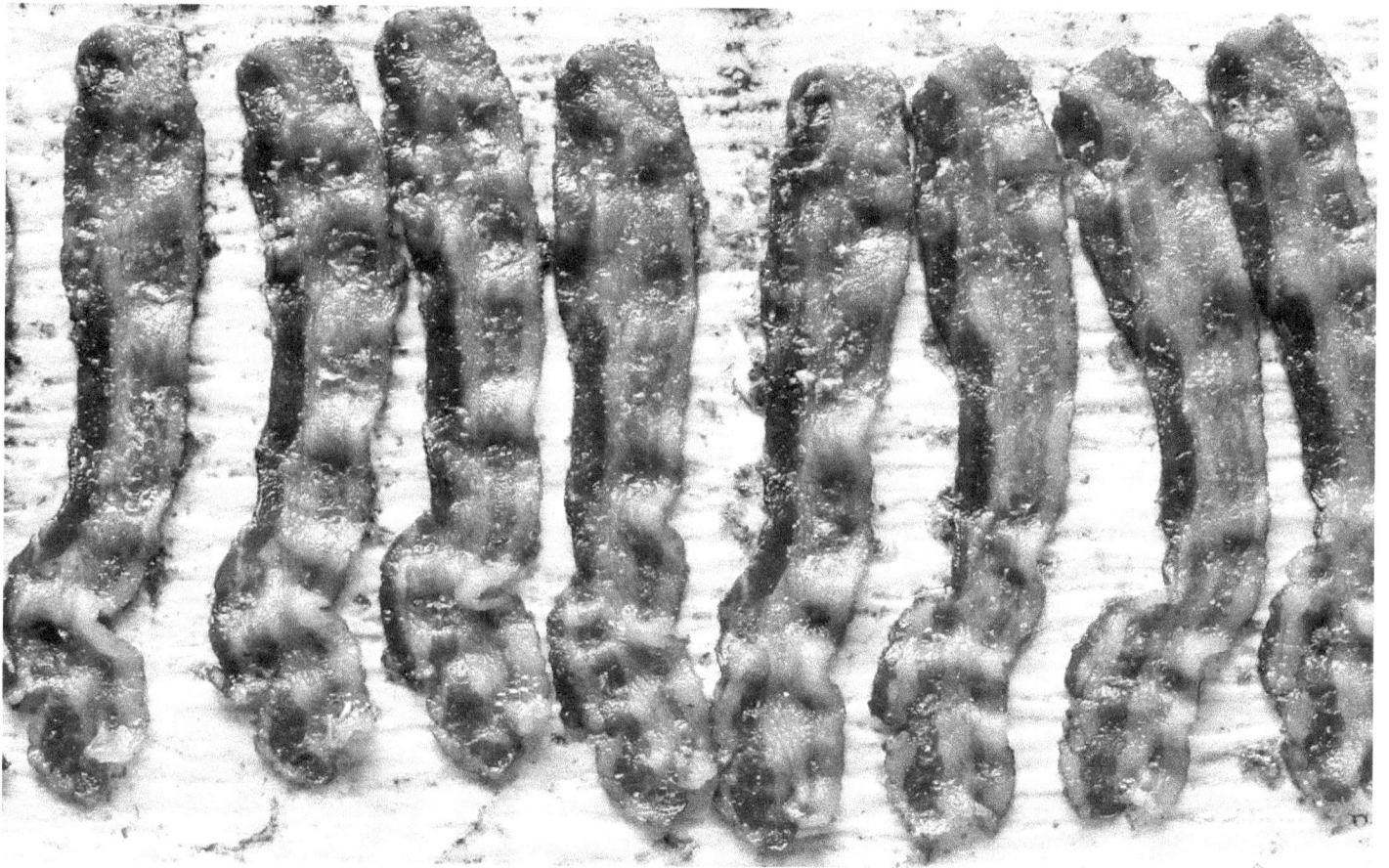

54 ROASTED LEEKS WITH EGGS

(Ready in about 40 minutes | Serving 2 | Difficulty: Easy)

Per serving: Kcal 1219, Fat: 124.6g, Net Carbs: 27.8g, Protein: 11.8g

Ingredients

- 3 green onions
- 2 leeks
- 2 tbsp. melted ghee (clarified butter)
- ¼ tsp. ground black pepper
- ½ tsp. sea salt

Avocado Vinaigrette:

- ¾ cup of light olive oil
- ⅛ tsp. red pepper flakes
- 1 ripe avocado, flesh scooped from the skin, pitted
- 1 lemon, juiced
- Ground black pepper and salt according to taste
- ¼ cup of red wine vinegar
- 1 tsp. olive oil
- ¼ cup of sliced, toasted almonds
- 2 eggs

Instructions

- Preheat oven to 400 degrees Fahrenheit.
- Green tops and bottom half-inch of the leeks should be discarded. Leeks can be sliced in half lengthwise.
- On a sheet tray, arrange the green onions and leeks. Drizzle ghee on top. Season with salt and pepper.
- For fifteen to twenty minutes in a preheated oven, roast till brown.

- In a food processor, thoroughly 3/4 cup olive oil, mix avocado, vinegar, lemon juice, pepper, and salt to make the vinaigrette

- In a skillet on medium-low flame, heat 1 tsp. oil for two to three minutes, or before whites are just set and the yolks are already runny, break eggs onto the opposite sides of the skillet.

- Remove the leeks and onions from the oven and put them on top with the sunny-side-up eggs. On top, sprinkle red pepper flakes and almonds. Finish with an avocado vinaigrette drizzle.

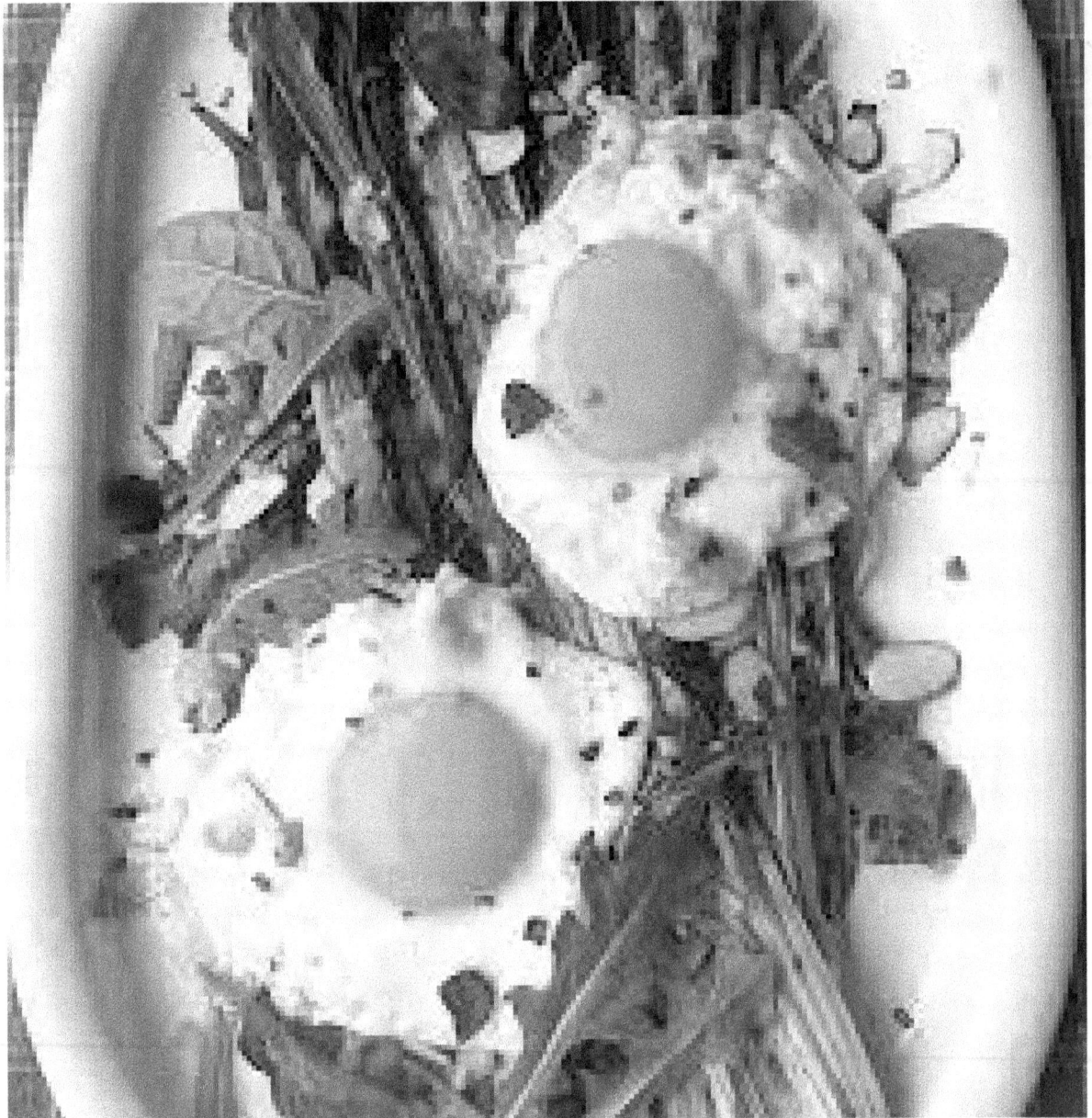

55 GLUTEN-FREE BAGELS

(Ready in about 30 minutes | Serving 6 | Difficulty: Easy)

Per serving: Kcal 364, Fat: 27.9g, Net Carbs: 9.7g, Protein: 20.9g

Ingredients

- 1 tbsp. baking powder, gluten-free
- 1 ½ cups of almond flour
- 2 eggs
- 1 tsp. garlic salt
- 2 oz. cream cheese, cubed
- 2 ½ cups of shredded mozzarella cheese

Instructions

- Preheat oven to 400 degrees Fahrenheit. Using parchment paper, line the baking sheet.
- In a mixing bowl, add the baking powder, garlic salt, and almond flour.
- In the microwave-safe bowl, mix mozzarella and cream cheese. Microwave for one minute, then remove and mix. Microwave for another minute, then take it off and stir until all is well combined. Working fast, stir the eggs and flour mixture into melted cheese mixture. Knead the dough by hand until it becomes a sticky dough. Continue kneading and pressing the dough for approximately two minutes or until it is fully uniform.
- The dough can be divided into six equal bits. Roll each one into the long log, then push the ends together to form a bagel shape and put it on the baking sheet that has been prepared.
- For ten to fourteen minutes in the preheated oven, bake till the bagels are golden.

55 KETO ZUCCHINI HASH

(Ready in about 30 minutes | Serving 4 | Difficulty: Easy)

Per serving: Kcal 200, Fat: 17.9g, Net Carbs: 5g, Protein: g

Ingredients

- 3 tbsp. coconut oil
- 4 small zucchini, squeezed dry and grated
- 1 tbsp. butter
- 1 tsp. chili powder, or according to taste
- ⅓ cup of grated Parmesan cheese
- 1 tsp. sea salt
- 2 eggs, beaten
- 1 tsp. cayenne pepper (Optional)

Directions

- In a small skillet over medium flame, combine the coconut oil, butter, and zucchini. Add the chili powder, Parmesan cheese, cayenne pepper, and salt to a mixing bowl. Stir until the cheese has melted.
- Reduce the heat to a minimum and whisk in the eggs before thoroughly combined. Adjust to medium heat and fry, stirring and tossing sometimes, for almost fifteen minutes, or till the edges of hash are lightly browned.

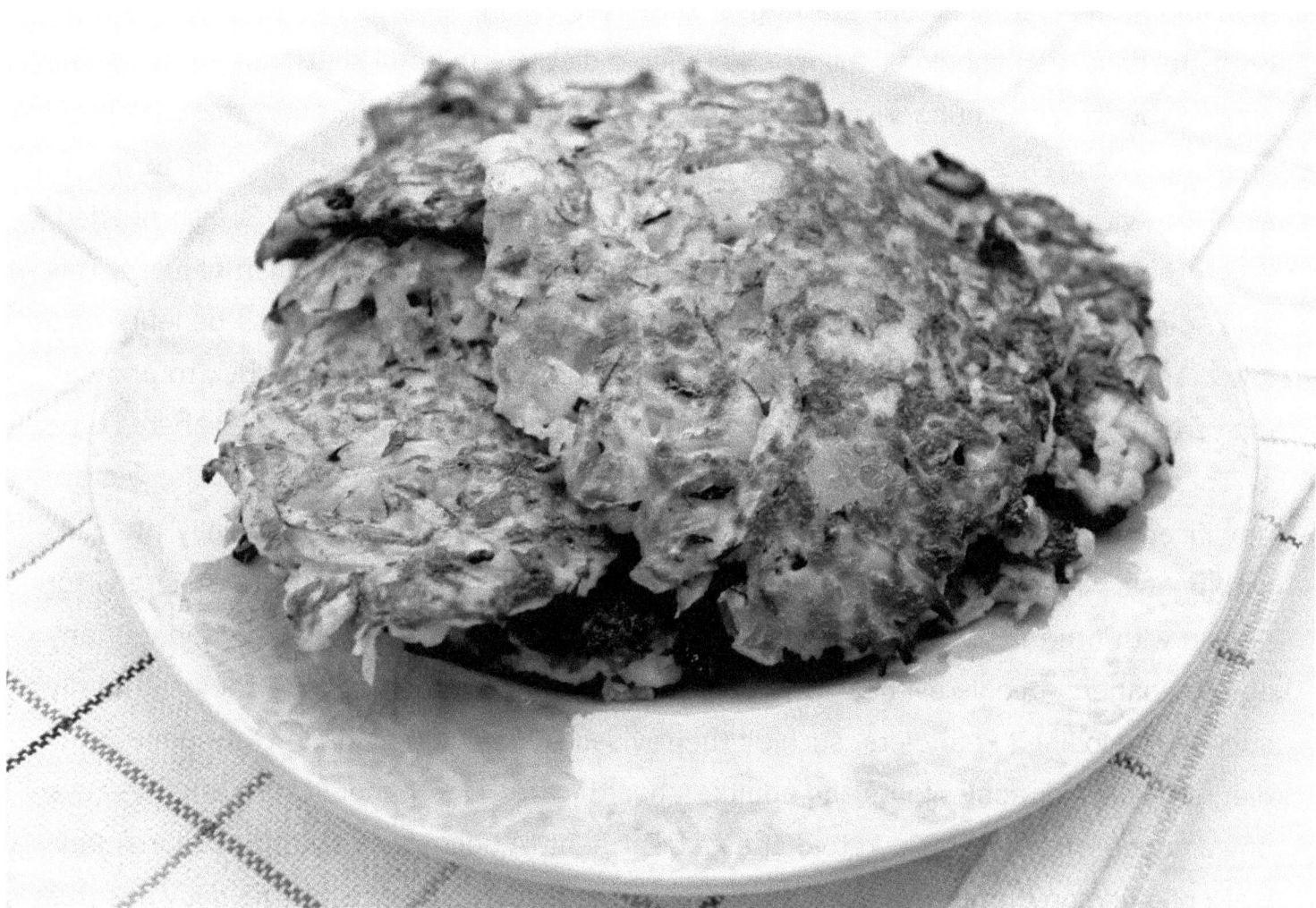

CONCLUSION

A keto diet may be a healthier option for certain people, although the amount of fat, carbohydrates, and protein prescribed varies from person to person. If you have diabetes, talk to the doctor before starting the diet because it would almost certainly need prescription changes and stronger blood sugar regulation. Are you taking drugs for high blood pressure? Before starting a keto diet again, talk to the doctor. If you're breastfeeding, you shouldn't follow a ketogenic diet. Be mindful that limiting carbs will render you irritable, hungry, and sleepy, among other things. However, this may be a one-time occurrence. Keep in mind that you can eat a balanced diet in order to obtain all of the vitamins and minerals you need. A sufficient amount of fiber is also needed. When the body begins to derive energy from accumulated fat rather than glucose, it is said to be in ketosis. Several trials have shown the powerful weight-loss benefits of a low-carb, or keto, diet. This diet, on the other hand, can be difficult to stick to and can exacerbate health issues in individuals who have certain disorders, such as diabetes type 1. The keto diet is suitable for the majority of citizens. Nonetheless, all major dietary modifications should be discussed with a dietitian or doctor. This is essentially the case with people who have inherent conditions. The keto diet may be an effective therapy for people with drug-resistant epilepsy. Though the diet may be beneficial to people of any age, teenagers, people over 50, and babies can profit the most because they can easily stick to it. Modified keto diets, such as the revised Atkins diet or the low-glycemic index diet, are safer for adolescents and adults. A health care worker should keep a careful eye on someone who is taking a keto diet as a treatment. A doctor and dietitian will maintain track of a person's progress, administer drugs, and test for side effects. The body absorbs fat and protein differently than it does carbohydrates. Carbohydrates have a high insulin reaction. The protein sensitivity to insulin is mild, and the quick insulin response is negligible. Insulin is a fat-producing and fat-conserving enzyme. If you wish to lose weight, consume as many eggs, chickens, fish, and birds as you want, satiate yourself with the fat, and then eat every vegetable that grows on the ground. Butter and coconut oil can be used instead of processed synthetic seed oils. You may be either a sugar or a fat burner, but not both.